KISS ME

KISS ME

How to raise your children with love

CARLOS GONZÁLEZ

Kiss me: How to raise your children with love

First published as *Bésame mucho* by Ediciones Planeta Madrid, S.A.
First published in English by Pinter & Martin Ltd 2012
This reprint edition published 2020

© Carlos González 2003, 2006, 2010, 2012, 2020

© Ediciones Planeta Madrid, S.A., Po de Recolets 4, Madrid 28001 (Spain)

Translated by Lorenza Garcia

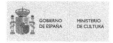 This work has been published with a subsidy from the Directorate General of Books, Archives and Libraries of the Spanish Ministry of Culture

ISBN 978-1-78066-313-5

British Library Cataloguing-in-Publication Data
A catalogue record for this book is available from the British Library

Pinter & Martin Ltd
Unit 803 Roach Road
4 Roach Road
London E3 2PH

www.pinterandmartin.com

CONTENTS

Acknowledgements

The author would like to thank Alicia Bair-Fassardi, Elena Garrido, Joana Guerrero, Rosa Jovè, Lourdes Martínez, Maribel Matilla, Pilar Serrano, Mónica Tesone, Eulalia Torras, Patricia Trautmann-Villalba and Silvia Wajnbuch for their invaluable commentary on the manuscript.

The testimonials from mothers quoted in this book are taken from letters to the author, mostly via the magazine *Ser Padres (Being Parents)*, and on Internet forums. Names have been changed to protect privacy.

About the author

Carlos González, a father of three, studied medicine at the Universidad Autónoma de Barcelona and trained as a paediatrician at the Hospital de Sant Joan de Déu. The founder and president of the Catalan Breastfeeding Association (ACPAM), he is an international lecturer on breastfeeding and parenting for health professionals and families, and writes for several parenting magazines. His books have been translated into 13 languages.

His books, *My Child Won't Eat* and *Breastfeeding Made Easy*, are also published by Pinter & Martin.

To Joana, Daniel, Sara and Marina,
who taught me how to be a father

FOREWORD

With our fast-paced lives and seemingly endless technological advances, it is easy to forget that at the heart of everything human beings have more basic needs – warmth, food and comfort. With every advancement it is also easy to forget that we are not some superior creature, but in fact mammals, albeit two legged ones. Importantly, our babies are born not with that fast-paced lifestyle in mind, but a fierce instinct to ensure those most basic mammalian needs are met.

Human babies are so vulnerable. Compare them to the baby giraffe or rhino who walks within hours of birth. Humans comparatively take much longer to even hold their head up let alone have similar levels of 'independence'. We are born so soon due to our extensive brain development meaning that the size of our heads impedes protection in the womb until we are more physically developed. We are born at a time when we must ensure our survival by convincing our parents to meet all our needs.

And our babies know this. They are programmed to want to stay close throughout the day and night. They are designed to protest at separation – after all, to them, they have no idea you are simply popping to the kitchen for a few moments. Their tiny tummies mean they must feed frequently, gaining not only energy but comfort from long feeding sessions. And we are wired to respond. Research has shown that we can easily identify our own baby's cry from others and find it far more distressing to listen to than a stranger's. Nature – and instinct – has programmed our babies to attach to us, and us to attach to them.

But we increasingly live in a society that will tell you all this is wrong. Babies, they say, need to learn to be independent. Babies, they warn, are just trying to manipulate you. Babies, they advise, should be taught to sleep and feed in a routine. Ignoring this advice and responding to that baby will create a 'rod for your own back', leaving you having to meet their needs forever more.

Or will it? Of course not. Copious research (and common sense) tells us that when a child has their needs met in a loving, timely and appropriate way that they in fact learn to trust. They learn that somebody cares and that the world is not a scary place. They grow in confidence and transfer that positive relationship to new ones, expecting interactions to be loving and caring and offering the same in return.

Responding to your baby or child in this way is not necessarily easy. Mothers and families need as much love and support as they themselves give to their child. But as this book will reassure you, one thing you do not have to worry about is the instinct and desire to respond to your child. Nor do you have to do this alone. This book will take you through each step and concern, exploring just how normal your child's needs to feed often, be held and sleep close to you are, and help open your eyes to your child's communication to you. It will show you how to model love, care and understanding to your child – and will stay with you as your child gains the confidence to in turn pay these forward.

Amy Brown
Professor of maternal and child public health

CHAPTER 1
The Good Little Boy and the Bad Little Boy

I have taken this title from Mark Twain's short story, not in order to speak, as he did, of two different children, but of each and every child, of children in general. Are children either good or bad? The reader will think: there are all kinds. Each child is different, and, as with grown ups, most are probably middling to good.

And yet, setting aside the merits of each child, many of us (parents, psychologists, teachers, paediatricians and the general public) have preconceived opinions as to the goodness or badness of children. We see them either as "angels" or "bullies"; when they cry they are either in pain or trying it on; they are either innocent or devious: they either need us or they manipulate us.

Whether we think of our children as friend or foe depends on this preconception. Some of us see children as gentle, delicate, helpless, loving and innocent; they need our care and attention in order to grow into wonderful people. Others see children as selfish, wicked, hostile, cruel, and calculating, and only by bending them to our will from the beginning, only by means of strict discipline can we lead them away from evil and make worthwhile human beings of them.

For centuries these two antagonistic visions of childhood have impregnated our culture. They are as prevalent in the advice of family members and neighbours as they are in the works of paediatricians, teachers and philosophers. The habitual consumers of parenting manuals are young, inexperienced parents (by the time they have their second child, they have usually lost faith in the experts and have less time for reading),

1

and they can find examples of both approaches: books on how to care for your children with love, and books on how to crush them. Unfortunately, the latter are far more prevalent, which is why I resolved to write this, a book in defence of children.

The stance of a book or of an expert is rarely explicit. On the back of every book it should state clearly: "This book assumes that children need our attention", or: "This book assumes that, given the slightest chance, all children will try it on." Paediatricians and child psychologists ought to provide similar explanations during the first appointment. That way, people would be aware of the different stances, and be able to evaluate or choose the book or expert most congenial with their own beliefs. Seeking the advice of a paediatrician without knowing whether he or she is an advocate of affection or discipline is as absurd as seeking the advice of a priest without knowing whether he is a Catholic or a Buddhist, or reading a book on economics without knowing whether the author is a Communist or a Capitalist.

Because, in the end, this is a matter of personal opinion, not of science. Although throughout this book I will try to provide arguments in order to back up my point of view, it must be said that, in the end, ideas on parenting, like political or religious ideas, are more about personal beliefs than rational arguments.

In fact, many experts, professionals and parents aren't even aware of these two tendencies, and therefore haven't stopped to think about which one they agree with. Parents read books that have totally different, often conflicting, views, all of which they believe and try to put into practice simultaneously. Many authors save them the trouble by producing a bizarre amalgam of the two approaches. These are the books that tell you holding your child is very good, but you should never pick him up when he cries because he will grow accustomed to it; a mother's milk is the best form of nourishment, but only for the first six months; mistreating a child is a very serious problem and a denial of his human rights, but a timely smack can work wonders... That is:

"freedom within limits".

We can see a classic example of this in the work of the educator Pedro de Alcántara García, who in 1909 quoted the philosopher Kant:

> Constant and extreme repression can be as damaging as continuous and excessive indulgence. Kant has said referring to this matter: "Children's desires should not be denied, rather they should be guided in such a way as to yield before natural obstacles – parents commonly make the mistake of refusing all of their children's demands. It is absurd to deny them the kindness they expect from their parents for no good reason. On the other hand, it is detrimental to yield to a child's every desire; doing so will doubtless preclude their ill humour, but it will also make them more demanding". Will should be trained, then, through exercise and restraint, both positively and negatively.[1]

Taken as a whole, these words appear fairly reasonable, and are not unfavourable towards the child (although the word "repression" jars a little in this day and age, doesn't it? We continue to repress children, while preferring to say we are shaping, educating, putting them on the right track). It depends on what we mean by "excessive indulgence". We all agree that, while we mustn't deny them things arbitrarily, if a child is about to jump out of the window, it is our duty to stop him.

But why do we evoke these restrictions when we speak of children? We would equally prevent an adult (whether our father, brother, spouse, boss or employee) from leaping out of a window, and yet this is so obvious when referring to adults that we don't see the need to mention it. Replace the word "child" with "wife" in the paragraph quoted above: "In a marriage constant and extreme repression can be as damaging as continual and excessive indulgence. It is detrimental to yield to a woman's every desire; doing so will doubtless preclude their ill-humour, but it will also make them more demanding."

In the space of two sentences, women have been described as demanding and ill-humoured. Isn't it infuriating?

For centuries husbands "naturally" dominated their wives, and similar things were written about women without anyone being shocked. No one would dare to speak about women in that way nowadays, and yet where children are concerned it is still acceptable.

Some readers may think I'm splitting hairs, making a meal out of this, taking Pedro de Alcántara's words out of context when in fact he was very respectful towards children. But there is more. A few pages later we read:

> In order to contain children's impulses and prevent them forming such habits, it is necessary to combat their desires, to oppose their whims, not to allow them to do whatever they want, or to be overly attentive towards them as many parents are.

We aren't talking here about preventing a child from playing with a gun, or from hitting another child, or from breaking a vase. This is about not allowing him to do what he wants "just because", for the pleasure of opposing him, when the author has just agreed that "it is absurd to deny [children] the kindness they expect for no good reason". Apparently, the author and his readers were unaware of any contradiction.

Many people are drawn to this type of woolly thinking, to the "yes, buts" and "no, buts", because the idea that extremes are bad and that moderation is a virtue is extremely common in today's society. But it isn't always the case. Virtue is often to be found in extremes. Here are a couple of examples, with which I trust my readers will agree: the police should never torture a suspect; a husband should never beat his wife. Does the use of "never" in either of these cases seem overly extreme, fanatical perhaps? Should there be an intermediary position, one towards which we might adopt a more conciliatory, understanding attitude, like for example only using a modicum of torture, or only torturing murderers and terrorists, or only beating a wife when she is unfaithful? No, definitely not. Good, in the same way, I am not prepared to accept that "a timely smack" is anything other than mistreatment, and I can think of no good reason for being attentive towards a child during the day but not during the night.

The book you are reading is not an attempt to strike "a happy medium"; it is taking a clear stand. This book assumes all children are essentially good, that their emotional needs are important and that we as parents owe them love, respect and attention. Those who disagree with these principles, who prefer to believe their child is a "little monster" and are looking for ways to bring him to heel, will – regrettably, in my opinion – find plenty of books more in line with their beliefs.

This book is in favour of children, but it shouldn't be taken to mean that it is hostile to parents, for it is precisely only in the theory of the "bad boy" that such a conflict exists. Those who attack children seem to think that by doing so they are defending parents ("a strict timetable to give you freedom, limits so your child doesn't try it on, discipline so he respects you, leaving him on his own so you can have some privacy…"), but they are mistaken, because parents and children are on the same side. Those who think children are wicked will likewise end up attacking parents: "You can't control him, you're spoiling him, you aren't sticking to the rules, you're weak…"

Parents have a natural tendency to believe their children are good, and to treat them with affection. One day, I arrived at my clinic early and was chatting to the receptionist. There was a mother waiting to see one of my colleagues. She had a two-month-old baby in a pram. The baby began to cry, and the mother tried to calm him by wheeling the pram around. As the baby's cries became more and more desperate, so the mother's pacing grew more and more frantic. When a child cries at the top of its lungs, minutes seem like hours. "What is she doing?", I thought, "Why doesn't she take the child out of the pram and hold him?" I waited and waited, but still the mother did nothing. Finally, although I have never liked giving unsolicited advice, I decided to drop a hint as tactfully as possible:

"What an angry baby! I think he needs a cuddle..."

At which the mother sprang forward and grasped the child (who instantly calmed down), before explaining:

"The thing is, you paediatricians say it isn't good to pick them up..."

She hadn't dared to pick up her child because there was a paediatrician in the room! I understood then how much power we doctors wield, and the pressures and anxieties a mother must go through every day.

I have heard the same explanation numerous times in less arresting circumstances: "I'd pick him up, only they say it gives them bad habits..." All mothers want to comfort their crying child, and will only be dissuaded if they are coerced or "brainwashed". And yet, I have never witnessed the opposite scenario: a mother spontaneously letting her child cry and only picking him up because she is obliged to ("I'd let him cry, but they say it can cause psychological problems...").

One-size-fits-all parenting

If there is an angel who records the sorrows of men as well as their sins, he knows how many and deep are the sorrows that spring from false ideas for which no man is culpable.
George Eliot, SILAS MARNER

Another frequent problem is that the advice offered in books and by experts is so vague it can be interpreted to mean almost anything.

I once went to listen to a psychologist give a half-hour talk to a group of parents. I didn't understand a word of what he said. In fact, I suspect he wasn't saying anything. When he had finished, everyone clapped. Consciously or unconsciously, some education experts appear to use methods similar to those of horoscope compilers: they give meaningless generalisations with which anyone can identify. If for example I say: "Geminis are affectionate and loyal, although they don't like being made a fool of", many Gemini readers will think I have described their personality perfectly. But what if I had said: "Sagittarians are affectionate and loyal...?" Another perfect reading. Of course, everyone likes to think of themselves as being more or less like that. No one admits to being unfriendly or disloyal, no one wants to be made a fool of.

In the same way, who would disagree with the following: "Parents should channel their child's potential, but without stifling his creativity"? The parents of six-year-olds Martha and Henry agree. Martha leaves for school at seven o'clock in the morning and arrives home at six or seven o'clock in the evening. She has lunch at school, and stays on after her lessons to do Spanish, computing and dance classes. A child-minder picks her up and looks after her until her parents get home. Henry's father has stopped working in order to look after his son. Henry has lunch at home, and has guitar lessons twice a week – not in order to kill time before his parents get home but because he likes playing the guitar.

Both Martha and Henry's parents think they are following the experts' advice to the letter: they are making every effort to channel their child's potential. But they are a little worried about this "stifling his creativity" thing. Aren't they inadvertently doing precisely that? Henry's father decides that from now on he will play basketball with his son as well as football (perhaps it's a mistake to focus on one sport); Martha's father decides to round off his daughter's education by signing her up for piano lessons twice a week from seven until eight o'clock in the evening.

Do you think Martha and Henry are receiving the same education?

These statements are sometimes so flexible it is possible to turn them around completely. If you liked: "Parents should channel their child's potential, but without stifling his creativity", how about: "Parents should allow their child's potential to flow freely, but they should set limits to his disordered creativity"? When you see these two sentences juxtaposed, it is obvious they are saying the exact opposite, and yet if you read one in one book and then a few months later the other in another, you couldn't be blamed for not noticing the difference.

And what about the following sentence: "The emotional bond between mother and child should be strong enough to make the child feel secure, but without becoming over-protective, in order not to stifle the development of his personality"? What does that mean? How strong is strong enough? How do you measure the strength of a bond? Is it possible to stifle the development of a personality? And if so, how? How can you tell when an adult's personality has been "stifled" as a child? When Isabel and Yolanda, who are both mothers, hear those words, they are a little concerned. Isabel's ten-month-old daughter spends nine hours a day at the nursery school and is fetched by her grandmother who looks after her from five o'clock until eight o'clock. Isabel suspects that her mother-in-law is spoiling and pampering the child. She wonders whether it might not be better to hire a child-minder to look after her for those few hours, before her young daughter's personality becomes completely stifled. Yolanda has taken leave off work in order to look after her ten-month-old son, who is breastfeeding, and who sleeps in his parent's bed. Last Tuesday she went to the hairdresser's, where she had to wait longer than usual, and when she arrived home her husband told her the boy had cried a lot. "Has the emotional bond between us been broken?", Yolanda wonders, "Will my son become insecure because of this separation? Should I have gone home when I saw how long the queue was, and had my hair cut another day?" Naturally, both Isabel and Yolanda agree completely with the expert in question; neither of them doubts the importance of a strong bond or the dangers of being over-protective.

Everyone can agree with these types of generalisation, because everyone can interpret them to suit their own ideas. A French-Canadian expert, Robert Langis[2] provides another example. In his book *How to Say No to Children* (a significant title in itself: children's biggest problem, apparently, is that they haven't been told "no" enough) he lists "thirteen ways in which today's parents are enslaved". These are very broad, the first, for example:

> We are unable to distinguish between our child's needs and his whims.

This can be interpreted in a hundred different ways. For some parents all of their child's demands are whims, with the exception of food. And food means exactly what is put on the table in front of her and nothing more, and she will have to eat at a fixed time and follow a strict code of table manners. For others, in contrast, what a child clearly needs is to be held most of the day, to sleep with her parents, to be cuddled and consoled when she cries, to eat whatever she likes and leave what she doesn't like, to play with lots of different, nice toys and to break the odd one from time to time. Yet these parents will all still agree on the difference between needs and whims; of course they aren't going to let their two-year-old child turn the gas on.

It is very easy to keep everyone happy with this type of general statement. In this book I will try to be more specific, albeit at the risk of disgruntling some readers.

The last taboo

> *What then is it in children that makes us*
> *so kiss, hug, and play with them [...]?*
> Erasmus, IN PRAISE OF FOLLY

Our society appears very tolerant because many things that were prohibited 100 years ago are now considered completely normal. And yet, on closer inspection, we will find there are also things that 100 years ago were normal and are now prohibited. So completely prohibited that it even seems normal to us, as normal as our great-grandparents' prohibitions and taboos seemed to them.

Many of the old taboos were about sex; many of the new ones are about the mother-child relationship, unfortunately for children and their mothers. For example, we use the word "vice" in a completely different way from our great-grandparents. Almost everything that was then considered a vice (drinking, smoking or gambling) is now treated as an illness (alcoholism, tobacco addiction, compulsive gambling), so that the sinner has become an innocent victim. Masturbation (the "solitary vice" that so concerned doctors and educators) is now thought of as normal. Homosexuality is simply a lifestyle. To speak of vice in any of these cases would be considered a serious insult. Today, only a few inoffensive habits of children are considered "vices", and in English they are spoken of as nothing more than "bad" habits: "He has the 'bad' habit of biting his fingernails." "He has got into the 'bad' habit of crying." "If you pick him up, he will develop a 'bad' habit." "He has got into the 'bad' habit of breastfeeding and won't eat baby food."

If you still have any doubts about what our society's real taboos are, imagine going to see your GP and describing one of the following scenarios:

1. "I have a little boy of three and I want to have an AIDS test

because I had sex with several strangers this summer."

2. "I have a little boy of three and I smoke twenty cigarettes a day."

3. "I have a little boy of three; I breastfeed him and he sleeps in our bed."

Which of these three scenarios do you think would elicit a reproach from your GP? In the first, he would say, "Ah, I see", and book you in for an AIDS test without batting an eyelid; at most he would politely remind you of the desirability of using a condom. Likewise, in the second he would explain that smoking is bad for your health (although, if your doctor is also a smoker, he probably wouldn't say a word). No one would give you a telling off: "How could you, a married woman, a mother!"

And in the third scenario? I can tell you a true story about that. When the psychologist at a nursery school discovered that Maribel was breastfeeding her sixteen-month-old son, she asked to see her in order to explain that if she didn't wean him immediately he would become a homosexual. (It is difficult to know which to be more surprised about, her prejudice against breastfeeding or against homosexuality.) As Maribel persisted in this "dangerous" behaviour, the psychologist rang up her home in order to speak directly to her husband and warn him about the harm his wife was causing their son.

Our society, which is very tolerant in some respects, is less so towards children and mothers. These modern taboos may be classified into three broad groups:

- With regard to crying: it is forbidden to pay attention to children, pick them up, or give them what they want when they cry.
- With regard to sleeping: it is forbidden to let children fall asleep while holding them or breastfeeding them, to sing to them or rock them in order to send them to sleep, to co-sleep with them.

- With regard to breastfeeding: it is forbidden to breastfeed them at any time or in any place, or to breastfeed a child when he is too "old".

Almost all of these taboos have one thing in common: they prohibit physical contact between mother and child. On the other hand, all activities that tend to reduce physical contact and increase the distance between mother and child are widely recommended:

- Leave the child alone in his room.
- Push him around in a buggy or in one of those unwieldy plastic carrycots.
- Take him to the nursery school as soon as possible, or leave him with the grandparents or better still with a childminder (grandmothers "spoil" children!).
- Send him off to summer camp as soon as possible and for as long as possible.
- Have "private time" as parents, go out without the children, enjoy life "as a couple".

Although some try to justify such recommendations by insisting they are "to help mothers to rest", the fact is they never prohibit tiring activities. No one ever says: "Don't do too much housework or he'll get into the bad habit of having a clean house", or "you'll have to go with him to do his washing when he leaves home." In fact, it is usually the most pleasurable part of motherhood that is prohibited: letting your child fall asleep in your arms, singing to him, enjoying him.

Perhaps that is why raising children is such a strain for some mothers. It entails less work than before (we have running water, washing machines, disposable nappies...), yet there are fewer compensations. In a normal situation, where a mother is at liberty to look after her child as she sees fit, the baby cries very little and when he does it pains her and she feels compassion ("Poor little thing, what's the matter?"). However, when they prohibit you from picking him up, sleeping with him, breastfeeding him, or comforting him, the child cries even more, and the mother is helpless in the face of this crying, and her response becomes angry and aggressive ("What's the matter with him now!").

All these taboos and prejudices make children cry, but they don't make their parents happy either. So whom do they make happy? Perhaps some of the paediatricians, psychologists, teachers and neighbours who recommend them? They have no right to tell you what to do or how to live your life or how to treat your child.

Too many families have sacrificed their own happiness and that of their children on the altar of a few unsubstantiated prejudices.

The aim of this book is to debunk myths, to break taboos, and to give every mother the freedom to enjoy motherhood the way she wants.

The road to ethical parenting

Lucky is the man upon whom his parents' kisses rained like manna from heaven!
Armando Palacio Valdés, TESTAMENTO LITERARIO

There is an old joke among paediatric students that goes as follows: "What are the similarities and the differences between paediatricians and vets?" They both have patients who can't talk, who don't come to see them of their own accord, and who are brought there by an adult. In both cases, the client (the one who decides to see the professional and who pays the fee) is different from the patient. But while the vet treats his patient with the main aim of satisfying his client, the paediatrician strives to find out what is best for his patient, even if this isn't what his client (the parents) wants. Or so it is at least in theory.

Our society doesn't treat children with the same respect as it does adults. When we speak of adults, ethical considerations are always fundamental and override effectiveness or usefulness. Compare the following two paragraphs:

OPTION A: When disciplining women, what is the difference between "reasonable" and "unreasonable" force? This contentious question was left unanswered in January when the Ontario Court of Appeal upheld a Criminal Code provision dating back to 1892 that allows husbands and employers to spank women for disciplinary purposes. The 3 judges refused to outlaw any particular forms of hitting. Instead, they recommended that husbands should not hit old women or women under 20 or use an object such as a belt or ruler when applying corporal punishment, and should avoid slapping or striking a woman's head.

OPTION B: When disciplining children, what is the difference between "reasonable" and "unreasonable" force? This contentious question was left unanswered in January when the Ontario Court of Appeal upheld a Criminal Code provision dating back to 1892 that allows parents and teachers to spank children for disciplinary purposes. The 3 judges refused to outlaw any particular forms of hitting. Instead, they recommended that caregivers should not hit a teenager or child under 2 or use an object such as a belt or ruler when applying corporal punishment, and should avoid slapping or striking a child's head.

One of the above texts is false; the other was published in 2002 in the *Canadian Medical Association Journal* (*CMAJ*).[3] Guess which?

The same article cites the arguments of those who are against corporal punishment:

. . . [there] appears to be a linear association between the frequency of slapping and spanking during childhood and a lifetime prevalence of anxiety disorder, alcohol abuse or dependence and externalizing problems.

And an expert adds:

[...] we are all looking for hard evidence on which to base any opinion or statement. But there isn't the kind of evidence we would like on this issue because it doesn't lend itself to randomized trials.

A randomised controlled trial (RCT) is where subjects are randomly allocated into two groups, which are given two different types of treatment. In contrast, in an observational study, the subjects do what they want. For example, you would like to find out whether exercise is good for backache. In order to carry out an observational study, you could interview people who exercise a lot at your local gym, and then interview 100 other people in the street or coming out of the cinema, who never exercise. Let us assume that people who do sport suffer less from backache. Is that because exercise is good for the back, or because people who suffer from backache never go to the gym? In order to answer that question you need to carry out a randomized trial. Find 200 twenty-year-olds, convince 100 of them to exercise every day and the other 100 not to do any exercise (this is the "control group") and wait five, ten or twenty years to find out which of them suffers more from backache. It is easy to see why RCTs are a lot more reliable, but they are also expensive and complicated to carry out.

What the Canadian expert is effectively saying is that, while we think beating children is bad because those who are beaten a lot become alcoholics and have mental problems, we can't be certain of this because no one has randomly divided 200 children into two groups, one of which receives regular beatings while the other doesn't, and seen what happens afterwards. And in the absence of RCTs, this could be a question of non-causal association, or there might even be an inverse causality (i.e., those children who as adults will become alcoholics and have mental problems are already badly behaved as children, and that is why their parents are "obliged" to beat them). And so it is possible, after all, that beating your children isn't such a bad thing, and at present we don't intend to make an official declaration against corporal punishment (by the way, why is beating an adult referred to as "domestic violence", while beating a child is referred to as "corporal punishment"?).

Apparently, beating children is only bad if it causes alcoholism and mental problems; in contrast, beating an adult is always bad, it is intrinsically bad. It is a crime, an abuse of human rights, whether it causes alcoholism or not. In fact, if beating an adult prevented alcoholism, it would still be bad, wouldn't it?

We would never permit employers to beat their employees, even if it increased production. We would never accept legalised torture, even if it led to a fall in crime. We would never impose on restaurants a single obligatory menu controlled by nutritionists, even if it reduced cholesterol. Firemen would never stop answering the telephone at night as a deterrent against people calling them out for no good reason.

No, not everything goes where the treatment of adults is concerned. Some things are done or not done on principle, regardless of whether they "work" or "don't work".

In this book I also argue for the existence of principles in our treatment of children, and that although certain methods may result in our children eating "better", sleeping longer, doing what they are told without complaining, or being quieter, we cannot use them. And this is not always because the methods are ineffectual or counterproductive, or because they can cause "psychological trauma". Some of the methods I will take issue with in this book are effective, and some might even be harmless. But there are things that simply aren't done.

CHAPTER 2
Why children are the way they are

No other people in the world love their children
as much or treat them as well.
Alvar Núñez Cabaza De Vaca, NAUFRAGIOS

Some people wish children came into the world with an instruction manual, or that those wanting to have children were forced to take a degree in parenting. Behind these apparently humorous statements lies the dangerous conviction that children cannot be properly raised without following the advice of today's experts. In fact, generally speaking, parents do a fairly good job, just as they have done for millions of years. Most of the mistakes they make don't originate from them, but from the advice of previous experts. It was doctors who, 100 years ago, recommended breastfeeding for ten minutes every four hours, which resulted in the almost complete failure of lactation. It was chemists who, many years ago, marketed a "teething powder" containing highly toxic mercury, to be administered to babies in order to help them to dribble freely, because "dribble retention" caused serious illnesses. It was doctors and educators who 200 years ago declared that masturbation "shrivelled the brain", and invented terrible punishments and complicated apparatuses to prevent children from touching themselves. It was experts who 500 years ago recommended swaddling infants to prevent them from crawling, because they had to learn to walk upright as opposed to crawling on all fours like animals. It is quite conceivable that all the mistakes we make as parents are an accumulation of centuries of misguided advice given by psychologists, doctors, priests and sorcerers. Thank goodness children don't come with instructions, and we don't need to take a degree in order to become parents!

How should a female rabbit raise her young? There is one easy way to find out: go into the countryside and watch any female rabbit. They all do it perfectly, in the best way their genes and their environment allow. They don't need to read an instruction manual; no one explains to them what they must do.

A female rabbit living in captivity will also raise her young perfectly, in the best way her precarious situation will allow. Her maternal behaviour is essentially genetically programmed. But for the bigger primates it isn't quite as simple; gorillas that are born and raised in captivity and have almost no contact with other gorillas, are incapable of looking after their young properly. They present abnormal behaviour that can result in the death of their young. Some zoos have resorted to putting young female gorillas in with older, more experienced ones, which are suckling, so that they can learn from them; or to showing them videos, or even to finding human mothers to breastfeed and look after their children for a few hours in front of the cages of pregnant gorillas.

And what about humans? What is the normal way to raise a human child? We only have to observe mothers living in the wild. The problem is there are no longer any human beings living "in the wild", that is to say, guided exclusively by instinct and biological imperatives. We all live "in captivity", that is to say, in artificial environments, and in human communities that conform to a set of cultural norms. Like the primates in the zoo, many of today's mothers seem to have lost the ability to raise their children instinctively. They have doubts, fears, they read books, seek expert advice . . . They even feel guilty when years later a new book or expert tells them to do the exact opposite. In the last 200 years, the way children are raised in

Europe has undergone radical, sometimes fluctuating changes that have affected the most fundamental aspects of parenting: how long should we breastfeed children, at what age should we feed them solids, where and how should we put them to bed, who should look after them twenty-four hours a day, what age should they begin school or nursery school, what clothes should they wear, where should they play, what rules should be inculcated into them and using which methods . . . ? Every new generation of parents has responded to these questions in a completely different way, and many of us no longer know how to respond at all. Did our great-grandparents get it right? Have we got it right? Or perhaps there is no "right" (in which case why worry so much about doing things "right"?). Or, worse still, perhaps we and our great-grandparents both got it wrong: we followed the arbitrary advice of false experts instead of doing what would be the normal thing for our species.

Undoubtedly, mothers 100,000 years ago didn't need books or experts in order to make the right decision at every moment; what a shame we couldn't be there to see it. Did they carry their children or push them around in prams? Did children sleep with their parents or in a separate bedroom? At what age did they stop breastfeeding? At what age did they begin to walk? What did mothers do when their children used swear words or quarrelled? How did they discipline them, how did they impose limits? We will never know. However, as bedrooms and prams didn't exist then, we can make a few informed guesses.

Because we have so little information about our ancestors, we are tempted to examine what we refer to as "primitive" societies. A long time ago, when I was nine or ten, I read in a picture book that Australian Aborigines never beat their children. That sentence stuck in my head, and has stayed with me ever since. No, my parents didn't beat me; but I had no idea why. Like many other children who read the adventures of comic book characters like the Spanish *Zipe y Zape* or listened to children's stories on the radio, I assumed that beating children was normal. In every episode Zipe and Zape, two young twins, would end up fleeing their parents, who chased after them with a slipper. The knowledge that it was possible to raise children differently, for an entire society to decide not to beat its children, not by accident or because they were never naughty, but on principle, was a complete revelation to me. I have just got up from my computer to go and find the picture book, which I haven't looked at for over thirty years, but which changed my life, my children's lives and possibly the lives of many Spanish readers. I quote:

> Aboriginal children have a good life, because no matter what difficulties their family group might be experiencing, they receive the most nourishing part of the food, and are always treated with great affection by their parents, who scold them when they are naughty, but never punish them.[4]

This is even better than I remembered! Aboriginal parents not only don't beat their children, they don't punish them either. I am far from being the first person to admire the way other cultures raise their children. In the quote at the beginning of this chapter, the sixteenth-century soldier and explorer Cabeza de Vaca wasn't referring to the cultured Aztecs or the powerful Incas, but to a ragged tribe of hungry, poor, disease-ridden Indians, who nevertheless welcomed dozens of Spaniards arriving in small boats from the Florida coast, without asking to see their documents, and shared the little they had with these illegal immigrants from Europe.

Is it a coincidence that children who are treated with affection seem to turn into more peaceable, kinder, more understanding individuals, who are also healthier and happier? You will find extensive information on the long-term benefits of affection in an excellent book, *The Tending Instinct* by Shelley E. Taylor.[5]

Naturally we aren't going to treat our children with affection "because it will make them more this or that. . .". We are going to treat them with affection because we love them, and, if they turn out to be more affectionate as a result, then so much the better. But we would treat them with equal affection even if they grew up to be unkind, because they are our children.

It would be a mistake to believe that "primitive societies" have the solution, because there is no such thing as primitive societies. All of today's societies are modern by definition. And, like ours, they all have thousands of years of history behind them.

There are hundreds of different human societies, and each raises its children in a different way. In many respects they all coincide: children feed from their mother's breast, their mother is their main carer, during their early years they are in almost constant physical contact with their mother or another person. It could be said that the ways in which most human societies coincide represents "normality" – the ways in which the first humans raised their children – and, in that case, we ought to be concerned that our modern, Westernised society is almost the only exception.

The Human Relations Area Files is an international organisation made up of universities and research centres from over thirty different countries. Its mission is to compile all the anthropological research documents, ranging from books and magazines to unpublished papers and notes, and it has at its disposal a million pages of information on 400 different societies past and present. Documents relating to sixty of these societies, from all five continents, have been included on an electronic database made up of 200,000 pages.

Some scientists made a detailed analysis of this database[6] in order to compare children from sixty different human societies (unfortunately the information is incomplete and in many instances some of the data is missing). In 25 out of the 29 societies where the relevant data was present, children co-slept with their parents. In 30 out of 30 mother's carried their children on their back. In none of the 27 societies where the relevant data was present did babies sleep in separate rooms, and only in 1 out of 24 were they placed in a separate room during the day. In 28 out of 29 societies, babies were always with someone or watched over by someone. In 48 out of 48, children were fed on demand. There was data on weaning age (complete cessation of breastfeeding) covering over 35 societies: before one year old in 2 of them; between the ages of one and two in 7 of them, between the ages of two and three in 14 of them, and over the age of three in 12 of them.

Virtually all societies agree on the basics; but customs such as food and dress are different in each culture, and I am sure many have found equally acceptable solutions to the issues of child rearing. Chimp behaviour is more varied and adaptable than that of rabbits; human behaviour is no doubt even more adaptable, and there are certainly many good ways to raise children.

Yet in some societies there are also long-established customs, certain types of tattooing or mutilation, for example, which are harmful to children. And I am sure many things in our society, like wearing shoes or learning to write, are beneficial, and there is no reason why we should relinquish them. No, the solution isn't to try to raise our children the way Bushmen or Inuit do.

As you can see, it won't be easy for us to decide on what is best for our children, on the normal way to raise a human being. We will need to observe how other mammals go about raising their young, in particular our cousins the primates. We will need to compare the way in which different human societies raise their children, and to choose what appears to work best. We will need to use our brains to try to figure out how our ancestors lived and why children are the way they are. And, above all, we will need to use our hearts: to look at our children and think about how to make them happy.

Natural selection and cultural selection

When our children take after us,
as they often do, they are our pride and joy.
Joan Manuel Serrat

Our children take after us, which is hardly surprising since they have inherited our genes. But from time to time a mistake occurs in the complex process of genetic copying and inheritance. This is known as a mutation.

Mutations occur randomly and we are all "mutants" in one way or another: our "mutations" usually involve minor chemical changes of no practical importance (a tiny, inconsequential alteration in DNA, or a slight change in a protein whose function remains unimpaired), and we don't even know they have happened. When a mutation is significant enough to produce an effect, in most cases this is harmful to the victim: a lion with poor eyesight, a fly with no wings... These animals die early, leaving few or no offspring, which means that natural selection tends to eliminate serious mutations.

Occasionally, the mutation has neither a positive nor a negative effect on the ability of the animal to reproduce or survive. Attributes such as blue or brown eyes, straight or curly hair are randomly distributed throughout the planet's population.

Very occasionally, a mutation can be advantageous to a living thing. A flower whose colours are more attractive to bees is more likely to be pollinated and to produce seeds. A gazelle that runs faster (perhaps because its muscles and bones are slightly different, or because its lungs and heart are bigger...) can escape more easily from lions. A giraffe with a longer neck can reach the leaves higher up on the tree when there are none left on the lower branches for its fellow giraffes. These animals and plants produce more children and grandchildren than their competitors, they are more "reproductively successful", and their genes will continue to be handed down.

Natural selection doesn't only determine our physique, it also determines our behaviour, insofar as it is instinctive – that is to say inherited as opposed to learned from our parents. A turtledove that doesn't incubate its eggs or protect its nest, a doe that doesn't constantly lick its young in order to remove the smells that might attract predators, are less likely to have offspring that survive and give them grandchildren. Over millions of years, each animal has evolved the type of behaviour that is most advantageous to its reproductive success.

But the behaviour that has evolved is "most advantageous" only within a certain set of conditions, of course. Firstly, the evolution of the "most advantageous" behaviour depends primarily on chance: rats could escape more easily from cats if, like bats, they had wings; but it seems the lengthy series of mutations necessary in order for them to grow wings didn't happen. Secondly, it depends on the characteristics of the animals themselves: it may be useful for a tiger to be more aggressive, but a rabbit is better off running away and hiding. A rabbit that confronted its predators wouldn't produce many offspring. There are even differences between the sexes: among birds, the male competes with other males to attract females and so has a more colourful plumage, while the female, which stays in the nest hatching her eggs, is more plain, for purposes of camouflage. The mutation that gives more colourful feathers would be beneficial to the male, but detrimental to the female. Thirdly, it depends on environmental conditions. Thick fur is good in the cold weather but not in a hot climate.

All these situations form the evolutionary environment of a species. And this environment can also change. A species that is perfectly adapted can all of a sudden find itself physically or behaviourally inadequate when confronted with changes in climate, vegetation, or the appearance of predators with new ways of hunting. If the change is slow and less intense, some mutations may occur that allow a species to change and create a new race or even a new species. In any event, the old species, as we knew it, will have become extinct.

Natural selection allows us to say that each animal looks after its young the best way it can. Over a period of millions of years, species that have nurtured their young more successfully have produced more offspring that survived, and natural selection has favoured that behaviour.

In human beings, and to a lesser extent in other primates, behaviour depends not only on genes but also on learning. Learned behaviour can be passed on both genetically and through example and education; not only to our offspring but also to other members of our species. This is what has enabled us to adapt to every type of environment, from jungles to deserts, from green pastures to landscapes permanently covered in ice. And it also enables us to adapt very swiftly to every type of change, because when someone discovers a solution to a specific problem they can pass it on to millions of people in a matter of years or even days, rather than to a handful of descendants over millennia.

When referring to natural selection among animals, figures of speech are commonly used which attribute freedom, volition and inevitability to what is simply a random process. You will often hear things like: "The male peacock has evolved big, brightly-coloured feathers in order to attract the attention of females", as if the peacock himself had designed and produced his plumage when in fact it is the result of a lengthy series of random mutations; and as if the female had nothing to do with the process. But there would be no point in the peacock strutting if the peahen didn't like it, and if peahens didn't show an instinctive interest in the feathers of their prospective mates – an interest that is also genetically transmitted).

Of course, no one really believes peacocks consciously produce their own feathers, everyone knows it is merely poetic licence (for scientists, too, have a heart). However, these figures of speech can be very confusing when referring to human behaviour, where natural selection has given way to cultural selection. For example, when a young man is said to "strut like a peacock" in his new sports car or jacket, evolution would seem to favour such behaviour because it increases reproductive success. Except that here the situation is very different. Firstly, because human beings do design and produce their own clothes for a specific purpose and not at random. Secondly, because that purpose may have nothing to do with reproductive success; moreover, it is probable that the young man who struts like a peacock has no interest in reproducing (rather in the steps leading up to it). Thirdly, because whatever its purpose, there is no guarantee that such behaviour will have the desired effect. A person may take great care over their clothes, their hairstyle, their "look", the way they talk and behave in order to attract the opposite sex, only to find themselves regarded as spoilt, conceited or downright ridiculous. And, despite their failure, others may still imitate their style, at least for a time.

Because of cultural selection we can no longer be sure we are bringing up our children in the best way we can. A particular innovation no longer has to contribute to our survival or that of our children in order to become widespread. Truth probably ends up imposing itself in the long term, but in the medium term (a few centuries), a whole society may do things that are harmful to children without realising it, convinced that what they are doing is irreproachable. There are plenty of examples in recent European history of mistakes that have been propagated by doctors and educators: there was a time when children were swaddled, or punished for trying to write with their left hand. Are we so conceited as to believe that we today are the ones who are doing everything right? Couldn't we be believing something, doing something, giving importance to something which in 100 years from now may puzzle, shock or amuse our great-grandchildren?

In other animals almost every type of behaviour is adaptive (that is to say, it contributes to survival). When we see a female animal doing something with its young, it is logical to think:

"There must be a good reason for it, otherwise she wouldn't be doing it." The first gazelle to spend all day licking its young didn't do it because she felt like it, because it suddenly occurred to her and she had nothing better to do; nor did she do it deliberately, thinking: "This way the lions won't smell my young." She did it because a mutation occurred that changed her behaviour: she had no choice in the matter. (I am simplifying, of course: it was no doubt the result of many complex mutations spanning millions of years.) And if gazelles continue to lick their young today, it is because that piece of behaviour was successful. In contrast, the first person to smack a child, to let him cry without picking him up, to breastfeed him on schedule, or to place a lucky charm round his neck did so because it occurred to them. This is voluntary behaviour, actions that aren't genetically determined. You can choose to do them or not. Perhaps the first person to beat their child did so by accident, because they were annoyed or incapable of controlling their anger, or perhaps they did it for a specific reason, which may have been for the child's own good, or for the good of his parents, or because some god willed it, or in accordance with a strange philosophical theory. Different families will often do the same things for different reasons. Some parents beat their son in order to punish him for fighting, believing he will learn how much being hit hurts, and that he has to be peace-loving; others beat their son in order to toughen him up, to turn him into an aggressive warrior who won't be dominated. Some parents hang a lucky-charm around their children's necks in order to keep them safe from evil, others do it to show they belong to a specific group, and others simply because they think it looks pretty. Some parents let their children cry because they think it does their lungs good, others to strengthen their character, others so they won't get their own way (that is to say, so they won't develop a strong personality).

And all of these innovations can spread, regardless of whether they work. The crucial thing is the ability of their inventors to convince the other parents. In the old days, a practice would spread more quickly if sorcerers or doctors advocated it; today selling books or appearing on TV can be more effective. It is even possible for behaviour that is detrimental to our survival or reproduction to appear and triumph. If drinking and taking drugs were hereditary and not learned behaviour, they would hardly have become so widespread (true, some people may be more genetically predisposed to addiction, but millions of smokers today aren't direct descendants of the first smoker, and it isn't genes that determine how much a society smokes, it is social pressure, health education, fashion or advertising).

Even when cultural changes are advantageous, they can clash with physical or behavioural characteristics which are the result of genetic heredity, and which cannot change overnight. Our diet allows us to live longer than our cave-dwelling ancestors, but with more tooth decay. The way we organise work allows us to be comfortable and to prosper, and yet we'd rather stay in bed on Monday mornings…

Consequently, when we see types of behaviour that are culturally, not genetically programmed, then the argument "If everyone does it, there must be a good reason", is no longer valid. It isn't valid for our society or for any other. Things cannot be justified by saying, "That's the way it's always been done", or "That's the way the Aborigines in Papua New Guinea do it."

How animals rear their young

Quick-witted or helpless?

> It is manifest to all that understand anything of children,
> that we are born into this world helpless.
> Daniel Defoe, MOLL FLANDERS

Insects, fish, reptiles and amphibians usually have innumerable young, which they abandon. Out of so many some are bound to survive. Birds and mammals, on the other hand, have few young, which they nurture, protect and feed while they are growing.

The degree of autonomy in newly-borns varies enormously among mammals. Many carnivores, like cats or wolves, have young that are helpless, scarcely able to walk and needing to be kept warm and hidden in a nest or lair. Small herbivores, like rabbits, also keep their young in a burrow, because the mother is able to stay in the same area for weeks, leaving the burrow to eat and coming back from time to time to suckle them.

Large herbivores, particularly those living in herds, quickly eat up all the grass where they live, and have to seek new pastures every day. Their young must be able to go with them from the very first day. That is why they usually have offspring that can walk and run within minutes of being born.

In her excellent book *A Natural History of Parenting*,[7] from which I have taken most of the information about how animals rear their young, Susan Allport says: "Predators – animals that are capable of protecting themselves and their young – can afford to give birth to helpless, sightless young."

And yet it seems to me herbivorous buffalo are able to protect their young rather better than carnivorous cats; and anyway, what harm would it do a tiger if her cubs were able to walk from birth? Even if she "can afford" to have helpless offspring, wouldn't autonomous ones be even better? I assume the answer lies in learning. The deer hasn't time to learn to run from predators. It must run immediately or be killed. Thus, it has an innate ability to run, which it will always do when faced with danger. Predators, on the other hand, chase their prey hundreds of times during their lives, and that enables them to learn from their mistakes, to perfect their technique, to invent new strategies to suit every terrain and every type of prey. A kitten begins chasing flies, balls of wool or its own tail; later on it accompanies its mother in order to learn the art of hunting from her; it will often practise by playing "cat and mouse" with its prey, releasing it then catching it again. A kitten might not be able to learn if it were "born knowing";

helplessness during the first few weeks of life is the price it pays for behaviour that isn't only genetic, but is also partly acquired through learning, and this makes it more adaptable to changes in the environment.

Primates are also helpless when they are born, probably because they have to adapt to living in trees. The Disney character *Bambi* (like all real fawns) falls flat on his face several times before he is able to walk; this doesn't matter at ground level, but it could be fatal if falling from a tree. Baby monkeys are helpless when they are born, and to begin with they move from tree to tree by clinging onto their mothers. Only when they have completely mastered the technique will they venture to do it on their own, without ever falling.

All newborn monkeys hold onto their mothers by themselves, with the exception of chimpanzees and gorillas, which are very similar to us and have to be carried for the first few weeks.

We are so like our cousins, the great apes, that we recognise ourselves in their behaviour and they in ours. They are able to learn from us and they can also teach us things. As we can see from this account given by Eva, a mother from Barcelona who was lucky enough to experience and recognise a magical moment:

We were on a visit to the zoo and we went over to the chimpanzees' cage. As we were watching them through a huge glass wall, our three-month-old son Xavi began to cry. A pair of chimpanzees came straight towards us and pressed their hands against the glass, trying to touch him. One of them was an old female, who, on seeing Xavi still upset, lifted her breast and offered her teat to my baby. Xavi stopped crying, and the female moved away from the glass, although she stayed close to it and kept trying to stroke him with her knuckles. When he began crying again, she offered him her teat once more. Besides feeling we had experienced something very special, I couldn't help being saddened by it. Two days ago, an old chimpanzee, forced to live in a zoo, had willingly offered her teat to a crying child that belonged to a different

species; six weeks ago, my baby started crying in a meeting, and most
of the people there insisted I shouldn't breastfeed him because he would
get into a bad habit, and that I should leave him in his pram (someone
even suggested he was anxious because he missed being in his cot…
Enough said).

Hide, carry, follow

Another basic difference is established between mammals that
hide their young in nests or burrows, like rabbits, and those
whose young go with them everywhere, either being carried
like primates, or following them like sheep.

The female rabbit spends as much time as she can at a few
yards from her burrow so as not to attract wolves with her smell
(her young give off a much fainter smell). Do you see what I
said? I'm using that poetic licence again, as if the female rabbit
were doing everything knowingly. She has no notion of smell, or
of wolves. She does what she does because her genes oblige her,
and because for millions of years, female rabbits whose genes
made them stay a few yards from their burrows have had more
offspring that survived than those whose genes made them stay
inside their burrows. The success of this behaviour proves that
it was useful in the evolutionary environment of the species,
that is, when there were wolves at large. Now that wolves
no longer exist in many countries, and there are scarcely any
other predators, this behaviour may no longer be evolutionarily
useful, but the rabbit continues to behave in the same way.

The female rabbit leaves her young hidden in the burrow
and only suckles them once or twice a day.[8] In order to be able
to survive hours without feeding, baby rabbits require highly
concentrated milk: 13% protein and 9% fat.[9] Kid goats follow their
mother everywhere and feed almost continuously, so her milk
contains only 2.9% protein and 4.5% fat.[10] (A human mother's
milk, incidentally, contains 0.9% protein and 4.2% fat. How long

do you think that allows a child to go without feeding?) Like an exquisite piece of choreography, the behaviour of mother and young and the composition of the mother's milk have all evolved in tandem: the baby rabbits that left the burrow and tried to follow their mother died early, as did the kids and lambs that waited for their mother instead of following her. Baby rabbits remain completely still and quiet when alone in their burrow, because crying out for their mother might attract wolves. In contrast, a kid goat that loses sight of its mother will immediately start to bleat frantically.

And so the behaviour of mother and young varies and is characteristic to each species; it is adapted to their way of life and needs. It would be absurd to try to explain to a female rabbit that in order to be a "good mother" she must spend more time with her children, in the same way that it would be absurd to tell a mother goat not to keep her kid "tied to her apron strings", because the kid needs to "become independent" and the mother "also needs some alone time with her spouse".

Primates in general need to be in constant contact with the mother. John Bowlby, an English child psychiatrist, describes in detail in his book, *Attachment*,[11] the bonding behaviour in different primates based on observations by many scientists. He describes, for example, the vicissitudes of a fellow researcher, Bolwig, who decided to raise an orphaned patas monkey, and become his surrogate mother in order to study his responses. Interestingly, as normal mothers do, he received advice from every quarter about the best way to bring up a monkey:

Bolwig describes the intense clinging shown by his little patas monkey after its caretaker had been persuaded (against his better judgement) to discipline it, for example by locking it out of the house or putting it in a cage. "Every time I tried … it resulted in a setback in the monkey's development. He became more clinging, more mischievous and more difficult."

Punishment and separation have the same harmful effect on monkeys as on children. See what happened when Bolwig shut his monkey in a cage:

> He would cling to me and refuse to leave me out of sight for the rest of the day. In the evening when asleep he would wake up with small shrieks and cling to me, showing all signs of terror when I tried to release his grip.[11]

If scientists were to discover a new, hitherto unknown animal, and wanted to find out quickly how it rears its young (without weeks of observation), a simple experiment would be to take their mother away from them. If they remained quiet then it would be normal for the young of that species to be left alone. If, on the other hand, they began to scream at the top of their lungs, then it would be normal for them to be with their mother at all times. And how does your child react when you leave her alone? What do you think is normal for our species?

Judging from our children's behaviour, from observing our closest (animal) cousins and from the composition of human milk, we can assume without a doubt that human beings belong to the group of animals that feed their young continuously. !Kung mothers from the Kalahari Desert in Southern Africa carry their young with them at all times; the children feed from their mothers' breast by themselves four times an hour or more for several years. Blurton-Jones, a British ethologist (a specialist in animal behaviour) who also studied the behaviour of children, suggested that "infant colic" could be a response to being fed at intervals instead of continuously.[7] In fact, it has been observed in baby macaques brought up in captivity and bottle-fed, that those fed every two hours suffer frequent vomiting and wind, compared to those that are continuously suckled by their mothers.

Susan Allport suggests that the change from continuous breastfeeding to breastfeeding at intervals happened very early, possibly with the beginnings of agriculture:

> [W]omen, even women who loved their infants dearly, must
> have leapt at the opportunity to put their babies down for a
> while in some safe spot – a house, a bed, the care of an older
> sibling – and go about their business unimpeded.[7]

This interpretation seems to me a little centred in twentieth-century American culture. Although the frequency of breastfeeding among the !Kung appears to be something of a world record, the truth is women still work with their child on their back in many agrarian societies, and feeding at regular intervals is a very modern invention. Many readers' grandparents (or great-grandparents) still carried their child with them wherever they went. The idea of scheduled breastfeeding is recent, and in the beginning the feeds weren't at three-, let alone four-hour intervals. As late as 1927, breastfeeding was recommended every two and a half hours during the first month.[12] It is possible to fool some people for a time, but most of humanity throughout most of history has breastfed on demand.

Moreover, I don't believe that most mothers have for thousands of years considered their children an "impediment", or that they "leapt" at the prospect of leaving them alone. I know many mothers who cherish their children more than anything in the world, and who feel sad (many use the word "guilty") when they have to leave them in order to go to work.

Millions of years ago, before the beginning of our cultural evolution, pre-human mothers already looked after their young. Both children and mothers showed an innate, instinctive behaviour, determined by their genes. That behaviour was perfectly adapted to the environment in which our species evolved, probably in small groups of foragers and scavengers on a plain inhabited by dangerous predators.

Since then, diverse human groups have invented new ways of raising children and have forgotten many of the old ways.

In traditional cultures, parents-to-be would learn by observing the "normal" way of raising children, and change was slow and infrequent. In today's society of information technology and uprootedness, a mother can reject her own mother's way of raising her as inadequate or old-fashioned, and replace it with advice from friends or things she has read in books or seen in films.

Accordingly very different ways of raising children exist side by side. Some parents co-sleep with their children while others put them in separate bedrooms. Some pick them up all the time while others leave them in their cots, even when they cry. Some tolerate their small children's tantrums and demands while others try to correct them using strict punishment. And there are hundreds of in-between ways, too, of course. Yet all the parents, with their different ways, believe they are doing what is best for their child, otherwise they wouldn't do it! And yet, regardless of what we have learned, read, seen, heard, believed or rejected throughout our life, our children are still born the same. They are born without having seen, heard, read, believed or rejected anything. At the moment they are born, their expectations aren't affected by cultural evolution, only by natural evolution, by their genes.

At the moment they are born, our children are fundamentally the same as the children born 100,000 years ago. In the last few thousand years, not to mention the last few decades, there have been huge cultural changes, and yet babies' behaviour has undergone no genetic changes worth mentioning. The spontaneous way babies behave, the way they expect to be treated, and their way of responding to the different treatment they receive hasn't changed in tens of thousands of years. As a baby grows, he begins to recognise and perhaps to accept the norms and customs of his culture. This is a gradual process that takes months, years. We cannot expect him to adapt instantaneously to our desires. If we wish to understand why children are the way they are, we must go back many thousands of years and look at the way we have adapted to our evolutionary environment.

In the lap of civilisation

Oh, God! to sail with such a heathen crew that
have small touch of human mothers in them!
Whelped somewhere by the sharkish sea.
Herman Melville, MOBY DICK

I deliberately avoided using the oft repeated heading "the cradle of civilisation", for as we know, in the beginning, there were no cradles.

They say our primitive pre-human ancestors began evolving into what we are today when they descended from the trees onto the plains. In theory, life on solid ground might once again have favoured more precocious, autonomous offspring. But before this happened, our ancestors had undergone another far more significant mutation, completely incompatible with precocity: intelligence.

On the one hand, intelligence requires learning (i.e., sophisticated behaviour capable of adapting to unpredictable circumstances as opposed to inflexible instinctive behaviour); and the greater the intelligence, the greater the time necessary for learning. On the other hand, intelligence requires a big brain, and yet to walk upright requires a narrow pelvis (if our pelvises were as wide as those of quadrupeds we would suffer from hernias; gravity would force our intestines through the hole). How can an ever-larger head pass through an ever-smaller pelvis? Birth became difficult. The ancient Hebrews seem to have understood the nature of the problem: "In pain you will bring forth your children" is the result of having tasted fruit from the tree of knowledge.

The head of a newborn cannot grow any bigger and so

evolution favoured a mutation that was completely new among mammals. We are born with half-finished brains, before the formation of the myelin sheath, the layer that surrounds the neurons and allows our nervous system to function. That is why our head is the part of our body that grows most after we are born, and why our offspring take much longer than any other mammal to learn to walk.

No other mammal requires feeding and protecting for so many years. A boy of nineteen living on his own, in his own house, with a job, would strike us as very precocious. But a fourteen-year-old boy living on his own would seem like a neglected child, and we would pity him. At what age do you think your children will fly the nest?

It is difficult for one person to take full responsibility for looking after, feeding and protecting children for such a long time. Mothers have needed the help of their family (father, grandmother, uncles and older siblings) and of society, the whole tribe. In almost all human societies, the father stays with the mother for years and helps her protect and feed her children.

This cooperation in child raising hasn't always been about carrying children or changing their nappies. In many societies and in many different eras, the physical care of small children is almost exclusively the task of mothers and other women. And yet fathers have continued to cooperate, hunting, protecting, or going to the office.[7] Even in the more male-chauvinist societies, a man who doesn't help support his family is frowned upon by his peers.

Why children don't like being left alone

And yet, no one managed to stem the distress and suffering of that unhappy child, whose mother failed to answer his call.
Fernan Caballero, LA NOCHE DE NAVIDAD

What would happen if a small child were left alone and naked in the jungle? After a few hours, the sun could scorch him or he could grow cold in the shade or be eaten by hyenas or simply by rats. Mothers who left their children alone for more than a few minutes soon had no children. Their genes were eliminated by natural selection. By contrast, the genes that compelled mothers to stay with their children were passed down to numerous descendants.

You are one of those descendants. Modern women have a natural genetic inclination to stay with their children. Langis[2] puts it very well, although in his ignorance he considers it one of "the thirteen ways in which today's parents are enslaved" (as if before "today" things would have been different, or as if doing what you want constituted enslavement):

We aren't inclined to leave our children in a stranger's hands...

Of course, this can be easily counteracted by more recent beliefs, opinions or customs, born of our cultural evolution. Mothers leave their children in order to go out to work, to go shopping, or to sit in front of the television. They leave them for a few minutes or for hours. They leave them with other family members, or with babysitters, or in nursery schools... But the genes are still there, and most mothers notice their effect.

The anxiety a mother suffers when she leaves her child appears over and over in sitcoms: the mother who wakes up in the middle of the night and goes to the baby's room to make sure she is still breathing, or who is going out to dinner with her husband and leaves a long list of instructions and emergency telephone numbers for the babysitter, then rings up endlessly from the restaurant.

I recently watched an American comedy film about a single mother, overwhelmed and stressed out by work. Her friend and psychiatrist convinces her to leave her child, of no more than a year old, with the baby-sitter and go away for the weekend on her own. Everyone around her mocks her concerns, her fear of leaving the child, her coming home early because he is running a slight temperature. Nobody in the film understands that having to leave her child every day in order to go out to work is precisely one of the main causes of her stress; nobody can even imagine a mother being able to spend a few relaxing days on holiday with her child. Insidiously, yet relentlessly, we are presented with cultural archetypes, we are told what is good and what is bad. In our society, leaving your children behind when you go on holiday is acceptable, whereas leaving your spouse behind is almost unthinkable. When you have a child, many claim that you have to maintain your "life as a couple", at least from time to time, and yet when you marry, nobody suggests you maintain your "life as a single person".

Many mothers feel bad when they leave their child at a nursery school, and for the first few days there may be as many tears outside the school as inside. "It breaks my heart to leave him", they explain. Many mothers feel bad when they go back to work. Society attributes this to "feeling guilty", and yet guilt isn't written in our genes, it is simply a cultural interpretation of an underlying phenomenon. For some this guilt serves a purpose. It would be uncomfortably subversive if a mother were to interpret her feelings not as guilt, but as anger or indignation at the inhumanity of our work practices or the inadequacy of our maternity leave (Swedish women have more than a year's maternity leave; Byelorussians[13] have three).

Why do children cry when you leave the room?

> *[…] produces in him a sudden feeling of terror, the same one we imagine grips the heart of a child when he is lost.*
> Charles Dickens, A TALE OF TWO CITIES

Immediacy is one of the characteristics of the infant's cry that shocks and upsets some people: "He screams bloody murder the moment he's left alone in his cot."

For some education experts, this is an unpleasant facet of children's nature, and all attempts must be made to combat their "egotism" or their "willfullness", to teach them to wait for their desires to be satisfied. Why can't they be more patient, why can't they wait just a little longer? We could understand if a quarter of an hour after their mother left, they became a little nervous, if after half an hour they began to cry a little, and if after two hours they were bawling their eyes out. We would think it logical and understandable. After all, isn't that the way we adults behave, and older children once we have "taught" them to be patient? But instead, our toddlers begin crying their little hearts out the moment they are separated from their mothers, they cry even louder after five minutes (as if that were possible!), and only stop when they are too exhausted to cry any more. It's illogical!

On the contrary. The immediacy of crying is "logical" behaviour, adaptive behaviour which natural selection has favoured for millions of years, because it promotes the survival of the individual. If in that tribe 100,000 years ago a baby began crying immediately with all its might, his mother would probably have picked him up instantaneously. Because that mother had no culture, no religion, no notion of concepts like "goodness", "charity", "duty" or "justice", she wasn't looking after her child because she thought it was her duty, or because she was afraid of going to prison or to hell. It was simply that her child's cries unleashed in her a strong, overwhelming impulse to go to him and calm him. But if a baby was quiet for fifteen minutes and then began to cry softly, and only began screaming at the top of his voice after two hours, his mother might already be too far away to hear him. This belated scream would be useless to his survival and would in fact probably hasten his end. Because, then as now, a child's anguished cry is music to the ears of hyenas.

And, if we think about it for a while, we will see that we

adults, when separated from a loved one, only behave in what we consider a "logical" and "understandable" way (becoming gradually "annoyed") once we are confident the missing person will return. Imagine your fifteen-year-old daughter is at school. During school hours being apart from her doesn't concern you in the slightest because you know perfectly well where she is and at what time she will be back. (Does your two-year-old son know where you are and when you will be back? Even if you could tell him, he wouldn't understand!) Imagine she is half an hour late, it will be simple to dispel your initial fears ("The bus is late, she's chatting with her friends, she's probably gone to buy a new pen..."). If another half hour goes by, you will start to get annoyed ("These kids, it's unbelievable, they're so thoughtless, she could at least have phoned, that's why I bought her a mobile phone..."). If she is two or three hours late, you will begin to phone her friends to see if she has gone to their houses. If she still isn't home five hours later, you will be crying and ringing the hospitals to see if she has been run over. Before twelve hours have elapsed you will be crying even more and will phone the police, who will explain to you that many teenagers go missing for any number of reasons, and that almost all of them come back within three days. During those three days you will cling to that hope. But you will be crying more and more, and by the end of a week you will be a living image of despair.

Now imagine you have a big row with your fifteen-year-old daughter in which hurtful words and accusations are bandied about, and finally she stuffs some clothes in a backpack and screams: "I hate you, I hate you all, I'm sick of this family, I'm leaving for good, I never want to see you again", and she goes out slamming the door behind her. How many hours will you wait, happy and nonchalant, before you start crying? Won't you be crying before she's even out the door, won't you follow her down the stairs, won't you run after her in the street, won't you try to grab her, oblivious to the spectacle you are making of yourself in full view of the neighbours, won't you kneel down before her and beg her not to go, won't you run after her until exhaustion prevents you from going any further? Would you consider yourself "infantile" or "egoistic" if you behaved like that? Do you think you would hear the neighbours say: "See what a spoilt mother she is, her daughter only left five minutes ago and she's already crying hysterically. I'm sure she does it to get attention"?

Yes, it is easy to be patient when you are convinced your loved one will come back. But you wouldn't be so patient if you were less sure. And when you are absolutely convinced your loved one isn't coming back, then of course you wouldn't show any patience at all.

There is no need to wait fifteen years to experience such a scene. Your daughter already behaves that way every time you leave her. Because she is still too young to know whether you will come back or not, or when you will come back, or how far away you will be in the meantime. And, as a fail-safe, her automatic, instinctive behaviour, inherited from her ancestors over thousands of years, will make her respond to the worst-case scenario. Every time you leave your daughter, she will cry as if you had gone forever (and what about mothers who try to "calm" their children by saying things like, "If you're bad, mummy will go away"; "If you're naughty, mummy won't love you anymore"?).

Within three, four, or five years, once she begins to understand that her mother will come back, your daughter will gradually be able to remain calmer for longer and longer periods. But not because she is "less egoistic" or "more understanding", and much less because you have "taught her to postpone the fulfilment of her desires" by following the advice given in a book.

Newborns need physical contact; it has been experimentally proven that during the first hour after birth, babies in their cots cry ten times more than those held in their mothers' arms.[14]

After a few months, they will probably be happy with simple eye contact. Your child will be happy, at least for a while, if he can see you and you smile at him and say things to him from time to time. A hundred thousand years ago, one-month-old babies were most likely never separated from their mothers, because that would have meant being left on the ground, naked. Nowadays they are wrapped up in a snug place, and although their instinct keeps telling them they would be better off in someone's arms, they are so understanding and want so much to please us that most will resign themselves to spending a few minutes in a chair. But the moment you leave your baby's field of vision, he will begin to "scream bloody murder". How many times have I heard mothers use this expression! Because, in fact, for thousands of years death was the fate of babies whose cries went unanswered.

Of course, the environment in which our children are raised today is very different from the one in which our species evolved. When you leave your child in his cot, you know he isn't going to get cold or hot, that the walls and the roof are protecting him from wind and rain, that he won't be eaten by wolves or rats, or stung by ants; you know you'll only be a few yards away in the room next door, and that you will go to him if there is the slightest problem. But your child doesn't know that. He cannot know it. He will respond in exactly the same way a Palaeolithic baby would have responded in the same situation. Not because he is afraid of wolves; he has no idea wolves even exist (or that they are becoming extinct). What he feels is panic at being left alone. His cries don't reflect real danger, but a situation – that of being left alone, which for thousands of years invariably meant danger. Babies cry when you leave them on their own, whether or not there is a threat of wolves.

So, will children be different thousands of years from now because of evolution? Will they no longer need to be with us, and be happy to be left alone? Probably not. Evolution happens over time, and yet time doesn't cause evolution. Mutations are needed, mutations that produce a selective advantage. If there are mutations and no advantage, millions of years can go by without anything changing. Of course there are differences in babies' behaviour; some cry desperately at being left alone for the briefest moment and others cry very little or not at all. In newborns these differences are genetic; after a few weeks, environment and experience begin to interact with the genetic makeup, changing babies' behaviour (babies in the West, who spend long periods in their cots cry much more than babies from other societies who are held most of the time). Let us suppose only 1% of babies never cry. If there is no evolutionary advantage to this, if babies who cry and babies who don't cry have the same number of descendants, in 10,000 years time there will still only be 1% of babies who don't cry. In order for this percentage to grow, in order for the number of babies who don't cry to increase to 5%, 15% or 80%, there would need to be a selective advantage: babies who cry would need to have a higher mortality rate, or the parents of babies who don't cry would need to decide to have more children. And this difference would have to be significant and remain unchanged for thousands of years.

As your baby grows older, he will begin to differentiate between situations where being left alone entails real danger and situations where it doesn't. He will be able to remain at home quietly while you go out shopping, but will burst into tears if he gets lost in the supermarket and thinks you have gone home without him.

Crying would be pointless if mothers weren't genetically programmed to respond to it. The sound of a baby crying elicits a powerful response in human adults. The mother, the father, even strangers feel moved, worried, anxious; they experience a strong urge to do something to comfort him: breastfeeding him, taking him out for a walk, changing his nappy, picking him up, putting more clothes on him, taking clothes off – anything to stop him crying. If he cries very loudly and relentlessly, they will take him to Casualty (and often with good reason).

When it is impossible to stop a baby crying, our impotence

can give way to irritation. This is what happens when we hear the neighbour's baby crying: social convention stops us from intervening, which makes it all the more annoying ("What are the parents thinking?" "Aren't they going to do something?" "The child is spoilt, our children never cry like that!"). Many neighbours criticise mothers whose children cry "too much", either behind their backs or to their faces, some even knock on the door to complain. More than once a mother has said to me: "My doctor told me to let him cry, that he's trying it on, but I can't because the neighbours complain." Even at the same decibel level, a baby crying upsets us more than a man drilling the road or a teenager listening to heavy metal music.

When parents are prevented from responding to their baby's cries in the most effective way (by holding him, rocking him, singing to him, or breastfeeding him) because of the absurd rules laid down by a few experts, what other solution is there? Can you leave your baby to cry while you try to watch television, prepare a meal, read a book or chat to your spouse? Can you listen to your own baby's cries getting louder, more persistent, more heart-rending, cries that pierce the "paper-thin" walls of some modern flats, and can go on for five, ten, thirty, ninety minutes? What about when he begins to make anguished noises as if he were choking or vomiting? Or when all of a sudden he stops crying, and far from feeling relieved you imagine he has stopped breathing, that he is turning white, then blue? Are parents permitted to run to his side then, or is that also prohibited because it would be "rewarding his tantrum"?

The other option is to try to calm him without picking him up, singing to him, rocking him or breastfeeding him. Why not with one arm tied behind your back, just to make it more difficult? Alternatively, you could put on the radio, pray, bribe him? An expert by the name of Dr Estivill suggests saying the following words to him (from at least three yards away, so he can't touch you):

"Mummy and daddy love you very much, darling, and they are trying to teach you to go to sleep. You sleep in here with Pepito, the poster and your dummy... See you in the morning."[15]

Loving words of comfort that will no doubt fill any baby's heart with serenity and calm, whatever the reason for his tears – from the age of six months! ("Pepito", of course, is a toy; don't imagine for a moment that he has a human being for company). Although, perhaps even Dr Estivill himself doesn't believe much in the calming effect of those words, since he advises parents to leave the room again as soon as they have uttered them, even if the baby continues crying or screaming (the ungrateful brat!).

In our country, as in many others, child abuse is a growing problem. Dozens of children die each year at the hands of their own parents, and many more suffer bruising, fractures and burns. Poverty, alcohol, drugs, unemployment and social marginalisation are undoubtedly some of the most significant causes of abuse. But there also needs to be a triggering factor. Why did they hit their child today and not yesterday? Crying is a common triggering factor. "He just wouldn't stop crying, it was driving me mad." What are parents supposed to do when the things that calm a child (breastfeeding, holding, singing, cuddling) are prohibited?

Responses to separation

> [...] as the little child knows nothing of parental love,
> but only knows one face and one lap towards which
> it stretches its arms for refuge and nurture.
> George Eliot, SILAS MARNER

In 1950, the United Nations (UN) commissioned John Bowlby to write a report on the needs of orphaned children. The result of his work is a book[16] examining the effects of separation on children, based mainly on the observation of hospitalized children, and on children from London who were separated from their parents during World War II (1939–45), and evacuated to the countryside to escape the air raids.

Among the frequent short-term effects of separation, the children exhibited the following responses:

- When the child's mother returns, he shows anger towards her or refuses to greet her and acts as if she weren't there.
- The child becomes demanding towards his mother or other carers; he constantly seeks attention, wants everything to be done just so, and suffers attacks of jealousy and terrible tantrums.
- The child relates to any adult who is present in a superficial though apparently cheerful way.
- Apathy, lack of interest in things, rhythmic behaviour (rocking movements), occasional head-banging.

In some cases, this rhythmic behaviour and head-banging can be normal, as explained by Dr Ferber (who was a great believer in training children to go to sleep by letting them cry for one minute, then three minutes, then five minutes; referred to elsewhere as the "Ferber method", in Spain this is known as the "Estivill method"):

Many children engage in some sort of repetitious, rhythmic behaviour at bedtime, after waking during the night or in the morning. They rock on all fours, roll their heads from side to side, bang their heads onto the pillows or mattresses. At night this may continue until they fall asleep, and in the morning it may persist until they are fully awake. [...] When rhythmic behaviours begin before eighteen months and disappear for the most part by the age of three or four, they are not usually a sign of emotional problems. Most often children with these habits are quite happy and healthy, with no discernible problems or significant tensions in their families.[17]

The double standard used here to measure what constitutes normal behaviour and what doesn't is remarkable. "Doctor, my daughter wakes up in the middle of the night…" "I see, she begins to cry and calls out to her parents. Your daughter is suffering from infantile insomnia as a result of learned bad habits; if this sleep disturbance isn't addressed in time, it may lead to serious psychological problems." "No, doctor, you don't understand. My daughter wakes up, but she doesn't cry or call out to anyone; she bangs her head against the wall." "Ah, well, why didn't you say so to begin with? If that's all it is, then there's no need to worry, head-banging is completely normal."

Returning to Bowlby we are reminded that some of the serious disturbances observed in children, who have been separated from their mothers and are in orphanages or hospitals, give a false appearance that all is well:

> A special note of warning must be sounded regarding the children who respond apathetically or by a cheerful undiscriminating friendliness, since people ignorant of the principles of mental health are habitually deceived by them. Often they are quiet, obedient, easy to manage, well-mannered and orderly, and physically healthy; many or them even appear happy. So long as they remain in the institution there is no obvious ground for concern, yet when they leave they go to pieces, and it is evident that their adjustment has a hollow quality and was not based on a real growth of personality.[11]

Fortunately, few children nowadays are kept in institutions such as hospitals or orphanages. But many are frequently separated from their mothers for several hours a day. The effect of this isn't as devastating, naturally, but similarities can be drawn. Some children appear "quiet, obedient, even happy" while they are at nursery school, yet begin to cry as soon as they leave. Or they appear to be perfectly accustomed to sleeping alone, yet "go to pieces" the moment there is a break in this routine isolation:

> It is enough for you to give in *once* to your child's demands (a drink of water, a song, holding her hand "for a moment", hugging her…) for you to have lost the battle: everything you have achieved ["training" the child to sleep on her own] will be lost.[15]

The most serious consequences occur after long separations lasting several days. But briefer separations also have an effect; in fact, the method psychologists use to determine whether the mother-child relationship is normal is the "strange situation experiment", in which a study is made of a child's responses to her mother leaving the room for three minutes.

The older the child, the less striking the effects of the separation, as Bowlby recalls:

> While there is reason to believe that all children under three, and a very large proportion between three and five suffer from deprivation, in the case of those between five and eight it is probably only a minority and the question arises – why some and not others?[11]

According to Bowlby, what makes some children better able to tolerate this separation is the relationship they have hitherto enjoyed with their mother, a relationship that causes an apparently inverse effect according to the child's age.

In children under three, the better their relationship with their mother the greater the effect on their behaviour after separation. Children who were mistreated or ignored at home, hardly cried when they were taken to the orphanage or hospital. That doesn't mean they are better at tolerating the loss, rather that they have less to lose. Their behaviour isn't normal for a healthy child of that age.

In contrast, children of between five and eight who had a stronger bond with their mother, who received more affection and were held more, are the ones who best tolerate being separated from her. The close contact they enjoyed during their early years has given them the necessary strength to tolerate hardship, what today's psychologists refer to as resilience.[18] Charles Dickens explained it very well a century and a half ago in *The Pickwick Papers*:

> He saw those who had been delicately nurtured, and tenderly brought up, cheerful under privations, and superior to suffering, that would have crushed many of a rougher grain, because they bore within their own bosoms the materials of happiness, contentment and peace.

Bowlby affirms that the emotional bond between mother and child is the template for all the emotional relationships we develop throughout the rest of our lives. This relationship with the mother then extends to the father, the siblings and other relatives; to friends, colleagues and teachers; to our own partners and children. He reached this conclusion not by studying adults and their hazy childhood memories, as many psychiatrists do, but from observing children and the young of other species.

Throughout this book I will make use of Bowlby's analogy between the mother-child relationship and other emotional bonds in order to explain some aspects of infant behaviour, but coming at it from the opposite direction. Much of the behaviour, which in children we happily attribute to "capriciousness", "play-acting" or being "spoilt", is deemed acceptable in adults. I should make it clear, however, that such analogies are purely didactic: what we know about children's behaviour comes not from observing adults and making deductions, but from directly observing children.

Imagine that you and your husband are at home one Sunday. Each of you is busy doing your own thing and pass each other half a dozen times in the corridor. Do you stop to greet or to embrace each other? Of course not. Most of the time you pass each other without looking up, without speaking.

Now imagine your husband pops out to buy something for

dessert. Doesn't he say, "See you", when he leaves, and, "I'm back", when he gets back? If he has only been out for a quarter of an hour or so, you may not even go to greet him, but instead carry on what you are doing and yell, "Hello", from the other end of the house.

The following day, your husband comes home from work. He has been away for nine hours. Don't you make an effort to go to the door to welcome him? Don't you give him a kiss (and expect one back)? Isn't the routine greeting a little more elaborate? Along the lines of:

"Hello, darling."

"Hello."

"How did it go?"

"Fine."

At that point, your husband will more or less leave you standing there and walk over to the television. For the first few months after you got married, you kept hoping for a longer exchange. But you have come to realise this is the way men are and you accept it.

Now imagine your husband has been to New York for a week on a business trip. When he returns, the usual exchange takes place:

"Hello, darling."

"Hello."

"How did it go?"

"Fine."

And he goes to watch the television… How do you respond? Are you going to let him get away with that?

"What do you mean, 'fine'? Is that all you have to say! What did you do? What did you see? Did you go up the Empire State Building? Did you buy me a present? How can you spend a week in New York and have nothing to tell me! Give me a kiss…! Don't you love me anymore?"

When two people who enjoy an emotional bond are separated, they both experience unease. In order to feel reassured, they need special physical and verbal contact (and sometimes further tokens of affection and attention such as a gift), and the longer the separation, the lengthier and more complex that contact will be. If one person refuses this reassuring contact, the other often responds in a hostile way. And, in the end, further words and further contact will be necessary in order to calm that person down (i.e. an apology).

The first example, passing each other in the corridor when you are both at home, requires no special contact, because there hasn't been a separation. Both of you were at home, consequently you were "together".

However, when it comes to a baby and her parents this changes. Going into another room constitutes a separation for the child because she doesn't know where her mother has gone. It will take her several years to understand that mummy is in another room and therefore hasn't "disappeared". And the dimensions are also different: to your daughter a few minutes seem like hours, a few hours seem like days or months and a few feet seem like miles.

Now you understand why your child starts crying when you leave the room, why when you go out to work or when she has been in hospital she wants you to hold her more and demands more attention, why when you pick her up from nursery school she insists on giving you a garbled account of everything she's been doing, and asks you to buy her things?

Sometimes, a child will ask for a sweet, an ice-cream or a toy because she wants it. Of course we aren't saying you should buy her everything she wants; that will depend on your finances, on her diet (i.e. how many ice-creams or sweets your daughter eats every week), on the number of toys she has and how often she plays with them. What I am saying in this book is that, if you decide not to give your child what she asks for, then let this be for a sensible reason (because she already has too many toys, because it is expensive, because sweets are bad for her teeth – and not simply in order to "train" her to "learn that she can't get her own way"; don't say "no" to your child simply out of spite.

There are other times when a child demands sweets or toys simply to try to "get attention". If, when she comes out of school, her parents don't show enough interest in her garbled account of everything she's been doing, and insist on correcting her speech instead of listening patiently; if they are sparing with their kisses and hugs, or even greet her in a hostile way ("Look at your dirty hands! Can't you wash them before you leave? Look at the state of your new skirt! And the buttons on your pinny! Do you think I've nothing better to do than sew buttons on all day?"), the child will probably demand everything she sees in the first shop window. She is asking for a sign of love. A misguided sign, because we show true love through respect, contact and understanding, not through presents and sweets.

For some parents it can be very tempting to give their children this false affection in the form of material goods. After all, time is money, but there are only twenty-four hours in a day. If you have money, it can be "cheaper" to buy your child a doll that can walk and talk than to play with her and her ordinary doll for an hour every day. This is the way we gradually "spoil" our children; by teaching them to value material things above other human beings. It isn't the simple accumulation of wealth that spoils them; rich children always have more than poor children, and yet some poor children are spoilt and some rich ones aren't. To spoil means precisely what it says: we "spoil" our children by not loving, cuddling, respecting and pampering them enough. It is impossible to spoil a child by giving her lots of attention, by cuddling her, consoling her, playing with her a lot.

We said that on Sundays, when you pass each other in the corridor, you don't need to greet each other because there hasn't been a separation. But if a couple were to spend an entire Sunday without talking to or looking at each other, without giving each other a kiss or a hug, wouldn't you assume they were about to get a divorce? Even when they are constantly in each other's company, two people who share an emotional bond occasionally need to do something together. If you forget this, your child will remind you.

He doesn't want to go to nursery school

In many everyday cases of separation, similar effects to those Bowlby describes can be seen, and mothers as well as experts continue misinterpreting the facts. Susana describes how her son responds to this separation:

Ramon started nursery school last week. He is nearly two and has never been before; well, except for two months last year... The problem is that since he started, from day two to be precise, he has been subjecting me to the most shameless emotional blackmail. And I am finding it "exhausting". He wakes up in a good mood, as always, eats his breakfast, watches the cartoons on the TV, and suddenly he starts repeating incessantly: "Mummy, nursery bad; mummy, nursery bad...", and he can go on like that for half an hour, with a sad look on his face, of course. On the way there he is fine, until he sees the nursery, then the real show begins: "Mummy walk; mummy pretty; mummy nursery bad; mummy kisses; mummy cuddles; mummy go home to sleep..." accompanied, of course, by crocodile tears and a long face... When his teacher picks him up, he begins to scream bloody murder; the poor little mite, how he cries, and I am almost in tears myself. I go home feeling awful. I feel really dreadful, I reassess the situation, I wonder whether I have done the right thing, I decide I have, I need time to find a job, it will do him good (this has been going on every day since last Monday). Well, at a quarter to one I am back at the nursery, to see if I can console the poor little mite, and what do I see? There he is playing quite happily with the other children. And his eyes aren't puffy so he can't have done much crying. But as soon as he sees me, he starts again, although with no tears this time: "mummy pretty; mummy home; mummy nursery bad..." Then his teacher tells me, laughing, that he hasn't cried all morning, and that the moment I left he began to calm down, and all he said was: "Where's mummy?" The same thing happens every day. At home in the afternoons he is terrible. He only wants to be with me, I can't even go to the toilet without him bursting into tears and calling me. If he wakes up in the night and his father goes to him, he says he wants mummy. If I go shopping I have to take him with me...

Ramon presents several responses which are typical in cases of separation: clinging to his mother and demanding her constant attention, appearing calm and cooperative while at the nursery, breaking down as soon as he leaves. Apparently it is precisely the fact that he doesn't cry when he as at the nursery that convinces his mother he is "putting it on". In order for this mother to accept that her son's suffering is real does he need to cry the whole time he is at the nursery? No one cries for that long. Human beings when faced with terrible trials and tribulations will cry for a while, then carry on. No one cries all the time, not at funerals, not in hospitals, not in prison, not in concentration camps. The fact that we stop crying, that we even try to "brazen it out", to face the situation with integrity, doesn't mean we aren't suffering.

We saw earlier how, among children under three, it is precisely those who enjoy a better relationship with their mother who suffer more when separated from her. Ramon's spectacular response shows us that he loves his mother very much, and that she has always treated him well. What a shame Susana can't see that!

The tragedy of this case is that the mother's misunderstanding can increase her child's suffering. Let us not fool ourselves: the ideal would be if she could wait a few more months before leaving him at the nursery school. But that isn't always possible; Susana needs to find work, and she has no choice but to leave her son at the nursery. No, this isn't the end of the world; it is a relatively brief separation, which can be compensated for. Ramon is explaining to his mother how to do this, how to heal his wound: he wants her to spend all afternoon with him, to go to him in the night when he calls her (I suspect he would probably like to sleep in her bed), to take him shopping with her, to give him lots of hugs and kisses. Susana could give him all these things and would feel better for doing so, because it would heal the wound she feels at being separated from him. But Ramon's teacher (supposedly an expert in child education) doesn't recognise the effects of separation on a child that age, and has laughed at his suffering. Susana has unfortunately chosen the opposite way: rather than acknowledge that her son is genuinely suffering, rather than hold him close to her and feel angry at the economic system that forces her to work when she has such a young child, she tries to convince herself that her son's suffering is play-acting, that his tears aren't real. Susana now feels anger towards her son, and accuses him of emotional blackmail. How will they salvage or compensate for what is lost?

Why does he always want to be carried?

Many women were nursing a baby, cradled in one arm,
and stirring a pot with the other.
Franz Kafka, THE TRIAL

Somewhere in Africa, 100,000 years ago, a group of human beings slowly crosses the plain. Perhaps they move in an almost military formation, like baboons: the women and children in the middle encircled by the men, some armed with clubs. A few of the women are pregnant, others are holding babies in their arms; the whole tribe moves at the pace of its slowest members. They stop here and there to pick fruit, dig up some roots or feed on some nutritious ants. If they are lucky, their intelligence, organisation and their skill at throwing stones will enable them to kill a few small animals or challenge hyenas for a piece of carrion.

And where are their babies? Did they leave them at home in their cot, with a baby-sitter, while they went out to work? Of course not. There were no houses or cots, the tribe moved as a group from place to place.

Baby monkeys clasp their mother's fur with their fingers and toes, and clench their mouths around her teat as she moves from tree to tree, securing themselves at these five points. Baby chimpanzees and gorillas are so similar to us that they are unable to cling to their mothers; she must hold them with one arm to prevent them from falling. But only for the first two or three weeks; after that they will hold on by themselves. How old would your child need to be before you dared leap from tree to tree holding on to him without the aid of a sling or a baby carrier? There is no other creature on the face of the planet that needs more than a year simply to be able to hold on to its mother.

Before there were such things as fabric and cord, not to mention prams, mothers held their children all day long, mostly in their left arm so they were free to eat with their right hand (or the other way around if the mother were left-handed). Their babies probably fed for short periods several times an hour, like those of the !Kung tribes today, (this intensive suckling suppresses ovulation, and the majority of mothers only bore a child every three or four years, unless one of her babies died young). When resting, the mother would sit her baby on her lap or would lie on the ground with him beside her. As he got older, the child needed his mother less and less and also grew heavier; the grandmother or the father or the older siblings probably helped the mother with carrying him. Babies were almost certainly in constant physical contact with others, most often with their mothers, day and night until they were able to crawl. And for a few years after that they remained in physical contact, if not day and night, then at least for a large part of the time. Even three- or four-year-olds, who can walk quite far, would have had to be carried if the tribe were travelling several miles.

And so, for millions of years natural evolution favoured children who demanded to be carried and who threw a tantrum when they were left alone. It was a question of survival.

Why won't children sleep on their own?

> *[...] the terror that grips children when they wake up in the night or when they are alone.*
> Alexandre Dumas, TWENTY YEARS AFTER

Where did babies sleep 100,000 years ago? There were no houses, no cots, and no clothes. No doubt they slept next to their mother, or on top of her, in a crude bed made of dead leaves. The father must have slept nearby, and the rest of the tribe no more than a few yards away. This was the only way for them to survive while they were asleep – the time when they were most vulnerable. The practice of husbands and wives sharing a bed is a throwback to those times, as is the unease (and sometimes downright insomnia) we adults often experience when a trip obliges us to sleep apart from our spouse. Many mothers, when their husbands are away, "let" their children sleep with them in their beds, and it isn't always easy to tell which of them finds the company more reassuring.

Can you imagine a baby, alone, naked, sleeping on the floor five or ten yards from its mother for six to eight hours at a time? It would never have survived. There had to be some means whereby the baby would be in constant contact with its mother, even at night, and again it is reciprocal: the mother wants to be with her child (yes, despite all the taboos about it, many mothers still want that), and the baby violently resists sleeping alone.

Sleeping alone! The chief aim of parenting in the twentieth century! As we have said, a child who didn't protest instantly when its mother left it alone on the ground awake, but which went to sleep, would have had little chance of surviving for more than a few hours. If such children existed, they would have died out thousands of years ago. (Well, not all of them, apparently some children do sleep through the night, instinctively and of their own accord. And if your child belongs to that category, don't worry, I am sure he is completely normal, too.) Our children are genetically predisposed to sleep in the company of others.

For animals, sleep is a perilous activity. Our genes compel·us to stay awake when we feel threatened, and to allow ourselves to drift into sleep only when we feel secure. We feel threatened in an unfamiliar place, and many people have difficulty sleeping in hotels because the bed "feels strange". We have difficulty sleeping when our partner is away or when we are in the presence of a stranger.

Imagine you have to change trains in an unfamiliar, distant town, but you have missed the last connection. It is two o'clock in the morning and everything is closed, so you have to wait in the station for the six o'clock train. Now imagine various possible situations: a) you are completely alone in the waiting room; b) you are travelling alone, but there are a dozen people in the waiting room, two families, a few elderly people, and a group of boy scouts; c) you are alone in the waiting room apart from five drunken skinheads; d) you are travelling with your husband and two other couples. Do you think you would fall asleep with the same ease in each of these situations?

Strangers in the night

Wheresoever she was, there was Eden.
Mark Twain, EVE'S DIARY

Javier is eighteen months old and a "bad sleeper". Every night he calls to his mother, Maria, asking for a story, for a drink of water, anything, and it has become an ordeal for the whole family.

They all say: "He's trying it on, just let him cry, there's nothing wrong with him." Today, Maria and Javier have gone to visit his grandparents in a remote village. The father is working and is unable to go. They have to change buses in a big town. However, the bus they have taken from the capital arrives several hours late. Maria and her son are the only people to get off the bus in the deserted bus station at one thirty at night. The local bus that goes to the village doesn't leave until seven-thirty the next morning. Mother and child find themselves alone in the poorly lit waiting room. The bus station is on the outskirts of the town, separated from the nearest residential streets by a few allotments, some warehouses and an industrial estate. Maria doesn't feel safe walking to the town. There is a petrol station next to the bus station; she will ask the man in charge to call a taxi, surely there's a hotel in the town. But has she enough money on her? She discovers to her horror that she only has just has enough for the bus fare, and she has forgotten her credit card. Well, never mind, she only has to wait six hours; she's better off staying where she is. The light from the petrol station reassures her. She would almost prefer to wait there, but it's cold outside.

Every now and then a car speeds past, or she hears a dog's bark coming from the industrial estate. At about three o'clock, five leather-jacketed bikers appear. They stop between the bus depot and the petrol station, and begin drinking beer, shouting and fighting. From time to time, one of them swaggers towards the bus station and urinates against a tree, while the others laugh and cheer him on ("Don't be an animal Paco, can't you see there's a lady present?" "Don't bother looking, madam, you won't see anything, it's too small!"). This goes on for an hour and a half.

Needless to say, Maria has spent the long hours awake on the chair nearest to the door, clinging to her son and their luggage. Javier, on the other hand, has spent the whole time asleep in her arms. Which of them is the "bad sleeper" now? In his mother's arms in a remote town surrounded by intimidating strangers, Javier feels safer than he does in his own house, in his own room, in his own cot. For a child of that age, mum is Supermum, the Invincible Protectress. Her lap is his home, his country, his Eden. Isn't that a wonderful feeling, mum?

In the Dark Ages

> *And if you have children, when they cry,*
> *does it not stir something deep inside you?*
> Victor Hugo, THE HUNCHBACK OF NOTRE-DAME

In that tribe we mentioned which lived 100,000 years ago, two mothers went to sleep with their children. We can't know how exactly, but we know what chimpanzees do now: when it gets dark, each adult makes a small bed of leaves and branches and goes to sleep on it. Male and female chimpanzees don't share a bed, they sleep apart (not very far apart, of course, as the whole group sleeps close together), but the mother chimpanzee sleeps with her offspring for the first five years.

In the middle of the night, those two primitive women woke up, and, for reasons unknown to us, they walked off leaving their children on the ground. One of the children was the type that wakes up every hour and a half, and the other was the type that sleeps through the night. Which do you think never woke up again? Or perhaps they both woke up, but one immediately began to cry, and the other only three hours later when he was hungry. Which child died of hunger? One began to cry immediately, and the other didn't make a sound until he was surprised by the appearance of a hyena. Which child did the hyena eat? One began to cry and he didn't stop until his mother came back to console him: he could have cried for half an hour, an hour, as long as necessary, until he was too exhausted to cry any longer. The other, in contrast, cried for a few minutes, and when no one came, he went back to sleep. Which of the two fell asleep never to wake up again?

Yes, you guessed right: our children are genetically programmed to wake up at intervals. Our children have inherited the genes of the survivors, those who triumph in the tough battle for life.

Babies don't sleep through the night, they have different sleep cycles during the night, like adults. The length of each cycle varies from less than twenty minutes to just over two hours; the average length for adults is about an hour and a half, and less than an hour for babies. Between each cycle we go through a stage of "partial wakefulness", which can easily become full wakefulness.

Even sleep experts, when they are "training children to sleep", acknowledge this;[15] their method isn't designed to prevent a child from waking up – that would be impossible. Their aim is for the child to remain calm when he wakes up and to go back to sleep without calling his parents.

Children are "on the alert" to make sure their mother hasn't left them. If a baby can smell his mother, touch her, hear her breathing, even suckle, he will go back to sleep immediately. Often when a baby feeds, neither the mother nor the child will wake up fully. But if the mother isn't there, the child will wake up fully and begin to cry. The longer he has been crying before his mother arrives, the more anxious and inconsolable he will be.

One planet, two worlds

> *"Who looks after these Milanese children, then, if they don't sleep with their parents?", he burst out, angrily.*
> Jose Luis Sampedro, THE ETRUSCAN SMILE

In some cultures, the practice of co-sleeping with your children is almost universal (and as a result sleep disturbances in children are almost unheard of). The psychologist Gilda Morelli and her colleagues[19] studied the behaviour and attitudes of fourteen Guatemalan mothers of Mayan Indian ethnicity and compared them with those of eighteen white American middle-class mothers.

All of the Mayan children (aged between two and twenty-two months) slept in the same bed as their mother, and eight of them slept with both their mother and father. In three cases fathers slept in the same room in a different bed (two of them with an older child), and in three cases the father was absent. In ten cases, there was another sibling sleeping in the same room, four of them in the same bed; four of the children didn't sleep with their siblings because they didn't have any.

The Mayan children stayed with their mothers who fed them on demand until the age of two or three, just before the birth of a baby brother or sister. The mothers usually didn't know whether their baby suckled or not during the night because they didn't wake up, and it wasn't something they seemed concerned about (in contrast, seventeen out of the eighteen American mothers had to wake up in the night to feed their children, most of them for about six months, and all seventeen of them complained that these night feeds were onerous).

Among the Maya there was no such thing as putting children to bed. Seven of them went to sleep at the same time as their parents, and the others fell asleep in somebody's arms. The ten who were still being breastfed fell asleep while they were feeding. No one told them bedtime stories, and they weren't given a bath before going to bed. Only one of the children slept with a doll; he was also the only one who hadn't slept with his mother continuously from birth, having spent a few months sleeping in a cot in the same room, before returning to his mother's bed.

The Mayan mothers couldn't imagine their children sleeping any other way. When they were told that American children sleep in a separate room, they responded with shock, disapproval and pity. One exclaimed: "But there's someone else with them, isn't there?" Co-sleeping isn't the result of poverty or of not having enough rooms, it is considered fundamental to the correct upbringing of the child. The Mayan mothers explained, for example, that in order to teach a baby of thirteen months not to touch certain things it was enough to say: "Don't touch it, it's no good, it could hurt you", and the child obeyed. When they learned that American children of the same age don't understand when they are told "no", or even do the exact opposite, one of the Mayan mothers suggested this behaviour might be due to the custom of separating children from parents at night.

It is fascinating to compare the way children are raised in different cultures. Meredith Small is the author of a key book on the subject, called *Our Babies, Ourselves*.[20]

Why is she waking up more than before?

There is always some naive soul who will explain to first-time parents: "Don't worry, it's only like this at the beginning; she'll start sleeping longer as she gets bigger".

How can she sleep any longer than she already does? Newborns already sleep more than sixteen hours a day; if they slept any longer, they would be comatose. We adults sleep more or less eight hours, and so at some point during our development we start sleeping less. "Of course", some might say, "they sleep fewer hours altogether, but they sleep for longer periods during the night."

This may be true in some cases; but for other babies it is the opposite. Let us see what Samantha says:

> *I have a baby girl of nearly six months old, whom I breastfeed (on demand). Up until now everything went smoothly; she would wake up a few times during the night, feed and go back to sleep (for three or*

four hours). But lately she's begun waking up every hour, hour and a half. She starts to cry without fully waking up, and, if I don't pick her up and breastfeed, she wakes up fully and it's much harder for her to go back to sleep. And so on every hour.

Laura is also six months old, and breastfed. Her mother tells a similar story:

When she was smaller, she would sleep for four or five hours in a row; of course for the first three months she almost never slept during the day because she had a lot of wind. Now she sleeps more during the day, at most two hours at a time, and at night she wakes up every two hours.

The same goes for Rosa, who breastfeeds her little girl:

Everything was going quite well, she was gaining weight and turning into a beautiful healthy baby. But since she reached four months old, we've noticed she only sleeps for a few hours during the night. At three months old she would sleep for over seven hours, from about nine at night until four in the morning. Now she barely manages to sleep for three or at most four hours.

These baby girls are all six months old, they are all breastfed, and they all wake up in the night more often than when they were first born. Is this a coincidence or could it be related to age and type of feeding?

The latter is probably the case. Researchers in America[21] studied sleep patterns in a group of children, and asked their mothers to fill in a series of questionnaires. All the children in the study had been breastfed for at least four months, but by aged two only half continued being breastfed.

They observed that whether the child woke up in the night or not depended on whether he continued being breastfed or had been weaned completely. The children who had been weaned slept for longer and longer periods: nine hours at a time at seven months old, then between nine and a half and ten hours up until they reached twenty-four months old. The children who were still being breastfed appeared to follow the same pattern: at two months old they were already sleeping six hours in a row, and at four months old, this increased to seven hours, but after they reached four months old, they began to wake up and, between the ages of seven and sixteen months old, they only slept for four hours in a row. At twenty months old they slept for seven hours, and it seemed they were at last beginning to sleep for longer, but this turned out to be a false alarm, and at twenty-four months old they only slept five hours at a stretch.

The total amount of sleep also varied; during the day the weaned children slept one or two more hours than those still being breastfed.

Many of the children still being breastfed slept with their mother, but began sleeping alone soon after they were weaned. Those children who slept with their mother woke up even more often during the night: at twenty-four months old, the children who were breastfed and slept with their mother slept almost five hours in a row; those who breastfed but slept on their own, almost seven hours, and those who were weaned and slept on their own, nine and a half hours. It is difficult to know whether they wake up sooner because they are with their mothers, or whether they are allowed to sleep with their mothers because they wake up, or whether they wake up anyway but the mother doesn't realise because they are in a different room. Most likely, it is a combination of all three.

According to diverse anthropological data and studies in comparative biology,[22] the normal period of lactation in human beings seems to be between two and a half, and seven years. A sample of American mothers attending nursing-mothers' support groups, who had been breastfeeding for more than six months, weaned their children on average at between two and a half, and three years old, while a few continued nursing their children until they were seven.[23] Therefore, those children who were weaned at four months old or at seven months old and began sleeping for longer periods, were breastfed less than the average and were sleeping longer than the average. It is the children who are breastfed who exhibit normal behaviour: waking up more frequently after four months old. That is what helped our ancestors to survive, by allowing children to be in continual contact with their mother. We don't know why children nursed with artificial baby milk have anomalous sleep patterns. The manufacturers of artificial baby milk keep trying to come up with a formula that will be "the next best thing to breast milk"; perhaps one day they may find a solution to the slight problem of children sleeping too long.

Some readers will be thinking: "Five hours! I wish our daughter slept anywhere near as long!" Well, remember this is only an average. Some babies slept more and others less (a strange law of nature decrees that it's always the neighbours' baby who sleeps longer). Moreover, the researchers didn't observe the children while they were sleeping, but rather questioned their mothers. Mothers aren't always aware of when their children wake up. By means of continuous ECG (electrocardiogram) monitoring and infrared filming, a colleague, Dr Jairo Osorno, discovered that when a child sleeps with his mother she is able to feed several times during the night while both she and her mother are still asleep. In the morning, the mother doesn't usually remember how many times her child has fed.

As children grow, they become more autonomous, more responsible for their own lives. In the beginning they are so helpless that the mother has to be responsible for maintaining this continuous contact, without which those prehistoric children, sleeping out in the open, would have perished within a few hours. What mother hasn't, at one time or another, gone "to make sure the baby is still breathing"? Of course she is still breathing, you know that, and perhaps your husband even laughed ("leave her be, she's asleep"); even so, you felt an urge to go and see your daughter because a powerful instinct prevented you from being able to spend so many hours away from your newborn baby.

Why "to make sure she's breathing"? Is this because mothers are worried about Sudden Infant Death Syndrome (SIDS)? No: SIDS has only become a subject for discussion in the media in the last few years. Long before that, countless mothers who had never heard of SIDS would go into their child's room, approach her cot, and gaze at her for a moment, smiling. This behaviour wasn't logical, it wasn't the result of a conscious thought process. And when they came back, if someone asked: "Is anything wrong? What made you go and check?", they would try to respond in a way that was culturally acceptable: "Oh, just to make sure she was still breathing". Because the true reason ("I don't know", "I just felt like it", "I missed her") may appear rather foolish. Other mothers living at other times and in other places no doubt offered different explanations: "I just went in to make sure he wasn't being strangled by a snake", "I was just opening the door to let in some fresh air" or "I was afraid someone might cast an evil eye on him." Even more mothers, living in many different places and at many different times, have never needed to invent such ingenious explanations, because their cultures didn't require them to be separated from their children at any time.

After a few months, the mother no longer feels this all-consuming desire to go and check on her baby every couple of hours. It is the baby who keeps watch day and night.

Her child is becoming autonomous. Now she is capable of keeping watch, of taking the initiative, of taking on responsibilities. You can sleep in peace now, in the knowledge that your baby will tell you when she needs you.

Co-sleeping in practice

There are some excellent books on co-sleeping, for example *Three in a Bed* by Deborah Jackson,[24] *The Family Bed* by Tine Thevenin[25] and *Nighttime Parenting* by William Sears.[26] I would also recommend a novel, *The Etruscan Smile,* by Jose Luis Sampedro,[27] as well as a short story, *Marc Just Couldn't Sleep,* by Gabriela Keselman and Noemi Villamuza.[28]

Some couples decide from the very beginning to have their baby sleep with them in their bed. Of course, the bigger the bed the more comfortable this is; but it can be done in a standard double.

Others prefer to place a cot with the rail down next to their bed. This can only be done if the two mattresses are flush with each other, and if there is no gap (in which the baby might get stuck and suffocate).

A single bed can also be attached to the double bed. This saves on furniture because the single bed can later be moved into another room with your child in it. The father can sleep in the single bed to avoid the danger of the baby falling between the two beds. If the beds are different heights, the legs can be unscrewed and the bed bases and mattresses placed directly on the floor; this prevents having to worry about baby falling out.

Another solution is to put the baby in a cot and take him into the big bed when he wakes up, to breastfeed him. If the baby falls asleep first, the mother can place him back in the cot. If the mother falls asleep first, the baby stays with her. It is usual for the mother to fall asleep first, unless she is making a special effort to stay awake. In which case she will stay awake, and, ironically, those mothers who put their child back in his carrycot in order to sleep better don't sleep as well.

Parents must take certain security measures. If the bed head has bars where the baby's head can get stuck, this should be covered temporarily with fabric. A baby shouldn't co-sleep with an adult who has been drinking or has taken sleeping pills, or who is severely obese (other than in these cases, there is no danger of the baby being crushed). Waterbeds and furry covers or rugs (natural and synthetic) should be avoided, as should heavy blankets and duvets, at least for the first six months (in winter it is preferable to turn up the heating and sleep with a summer duvet). It is important that the sheets don't cover the baby's head. And refrain from smoking: tobacco increases the risk of SIDS.

Never fall asleep with a baby on a sofa. There are too many places where the baby can become trapped.[29]

A radical solution to problems of space is the Japanese way of sleeping: directly on the floor on a futon.

When a baby sleeps with his mother, calmed by his mother's presence, he sometimes wakes up and falls asleep again without making a sound, and sometimes he will feed. The mother doesn't usually wake up and remembers nothing about it the following day.

Yet some families are driven to distraction because not only does their child wake up and feed, he screams and cries and demands to be picked up and carried around or sung to five or ten times during the night. This is normal for a few nights if the child is unwell, if something is hurting him or his nose is blocked, but for a healthy child it makes no sense to behave like that night after night. In our prehistoric tribe, children had to be as quiet as possible during the night because their cries would attract lions. So why do some children behave like this?

It may be because they have been made to sleep on their own for a time. If you have let your child cry in the night, and after reading this book you decide to let him sleep with you in the big bed, don't expect everything to go smoothly from day one. As we saw earlier, the normal response to being separated is for your child to be mistrustful, demanding and tearful for a few days or even weeks. You have to be patient, and give him plenty of cuddles until he feels secure again.

Yet I have also heard tales of children who, despite co-sleeping with their parents from day one, spend the night crying and unable to settle. Most parents would prefer not to have to get out of bed during the night, so before you do so you must ask yourselves if this is what your baby is actually demanding. Children sometimes make little whimpering noises when they are half asleep, and when this happens it is best to do nothing so as not to wake them up completely. Or they may start to gripe a little, and often it is enough to touch them and say "coochie coo" for them to calm down again. When the child is awake, but not crying, you needn't do anything to get him to sleep. Go to sleep yourself and let him do what he wants. Don't turn on the light, don't talk, and only get up if these softer approaches have failed.

When a child has got into the habit of crying until he is taken into the corridor for a little turn, it might be a good idea if dad does that and mum stays in bed. Most children prefer to be in bed with mum than carried around by dad (this is hard for the male ego to accept, but it's true).

At what age will she starting sleeping on her own?

This is a difficult question. Our society's attitude to co-sleeping is so negative that no serious study has been done to find out what the normal age is.

If nobody forced their children out of the parental bed, sooner or later they would end up going of their own accord. I don't know at what age, because I don't know anyone who has tried this experiment; the age would no doubt differ for each family, depending on the temperament and desires of the child and her parents. However, I think I can reasonably assume that none of my readers have, at this point in time, the slightest desire to go back to sleeping every night sandwiched between their mother and father. Japanese children commonly sleep with their parents until they are five, but this is a cultural issue, and needn't be considered "the norm". Chimpanzees also sleep with their mother until they are five, but chimpanzees reach puberty at seven, so that five years for them is equivalent to ten years for us.

When there were no houses and clothes, it is difficult to imagine a child under ten years old sleeping on his own. But now there is less risk involved, and many parents would prefer their children to start sleeping in their own bed before they are ten. Others don't mind co-sleeping or they like it. Since it does nobody any harm, they are at liberty to carry on co-sleeping as long as they want.

When children understand rationally that they aren't in any danger, that their parents are in the room next door, and will come if they need them, they are able to sleep on their own without crying, and to refrain from calling them unless some other problem arises. And yet their instinct keeps telling them otherwise.

Imagine you say to your husband: "Darling, since we aren't planning to have more children, I think it best that we stop having sex altogether." Rationally, he would understand this, but would he be capable of doing it?

In my own experience, and that of other families who practise co-sleeping, if towards the age of three or four you begin skilfully to sell them the idea ("Now you're bigger, you can have a bed of your own, and a toy cupboard…"), children will by and large accept to sleep on their own. But they will ask you to tell them stories and insist you stay with them until they fall asleep, and this will go on every night until they are seven or eight. And they won't want just anyone to stay with them, they will usually ask for their mother. It is quite typical for a father to tell a bedtime story, and another and another, and when at last he says: "Right, enough stories, time to go to sleep", the child will say: "I want mummy." And what mother hasn't, at one time or another, heard a little voice call out: "Mummy, mummy, come here, daddy's fallen asleep"?

Moving into a room of their own is easier if they share it with an older sibling. Although, at a certain age the older sibling will no doubt want a room of her own.

During the conflictive years, between three and ten, when reason (and their parents) tells them they are big enough to sleep on their own, yet their instinct draws them to their mother, children can behave in strange ways. They may call their mother, and be overjoyed when she comes, or they may be quite content just to hear her say: "Go on, go to sleep, it's late."

Pilar, who is ten, went through a phase of getting up five minutes after being put to bed, and climbing into bed with her parents:

"I can't get to sleeeep."

"Have you tried lying still and being quiet?"

"No."

"Well, try."

And she would go back to her room. A few days later, she had learned the routine.

"I can't get to sleeeep."

"Have you tried lying still and being quiet?"

"Yes."

"How long?"

"Not very long."

"Well try again for longer."

A few days later, there was no need to elaborate.

"I can't get to sleeeep."

"Do you know what I'm going to say?"

And Pilar would go back to bed. Some nights, if her mother wasn't too tired herself, she would go and spend a few moments with her. A few weeks later, Pilar began going to bed without any fuss; and, of course, her mother missed those moments.

Why do children demand our attention?

> "Mother! They're coming! Protect me!"
> "Yes, my darling, I will protect you."
> Victor Hugo, THE HUNCHBACK OF NOTRE-DAME

Some of us go to the park to watch the birds or the squirrels. But watching children can often prove far more rewarding. Indeed, going to parks and watching children ought to be a compulsory exercise for expecting parents. If you are already a parent, you are still in time to watch your own or others' children.

Let us watch the complex interactions of young children. You see a mother pushing her baby in a pram. She bumps into a friend. Approach discreetly and watch closely. Before greeting the mother, the friend (a woman – men are usually more shy with babies), will start talking to the baby. First she bends over until she is almost level with the child, her face inches from his, then she looks straight at him, smiles, and in a loud sing-song voice begins to make the appropriate noises ("What a beautiful boy", and "How is my little prince", although the actual words don't matter, and some people will stick to the usual "coochie coo!").

At this point, the child will respond (if he's in the mood) by opening his eyes, gazing at the intruder, pulling a face that more or less resembles a smile, nodding his head, and saying: "gaga" or some other baby word. From then on, the child will probably steer the conversation, while the nice woman limits herself to smiling back at him or repeating the word "gaga" or nodding her head, while the baby in turn imitates her imitating him, and so on.

Now see what happens next. The nice woman tires of this little game, and she begins talking to the baby's mother. The two women turn to face each other, and neither takes any notice of the baby. But you, as a casual, discreet observer, will have your eyes glued on him. You will witness a common yet little known episode in the lives of babies, one which the mother and her friend will be unaware of at that moment, because, unlike you, they aren't looking. You will see the baby try once, and then again, to nod its head, say "gaga" and smile. You will see his smile turn into a very different expression, firstly of incomprehension, then of unease, and soon of deep distress. Age and ability permitting, the child may try to repeat the word "gaga" in a more forceful voice, turn his head and his whole body in an attempt to find the person who has just vanished from his field of vision, jiggle the pram or throw away a toy to draw their attention. If at this point the mother or her friend say something friendly to the baby, he will immediately calm down (for a few seconds); if they ignore him, he may begin to whimper, then scream or cry his eyes out.

Why does he do this? Most explanations, whether coming from books or from "popular wisdom", are quite negative towards the child. They accuse him of being spoilt (but, if you are a tireless observer, you will see that all babies behave in the same way regardless of whether they are spoilt). They say he is jealous, which is one way of looking at it, although perhaps not the most appropriate. Is he jealous of the woman for talking to his mother, or of his mother for talking to the other woman? Imagine if you are sitting in a café with your husband and a stranger comes up, says "Hello" to you and makes some remark about the weather, then sits down and starts talking to your husband. For two hours this person and your husband sit face-to-face talking, without saying a word to you or even looking at you. How would you feel? If the person in question were a dazzling blonde showing a lot of cleavage, you might think you were "jealous". Yet if it were an old man with a grey beard, you wouldn't feel much better either. It would be closer to the truth to say that you feel "left out" or "ignored", and this is hurtful at any age. ("But in your example my husband has ignored me for two hours, whereas the baby begins to cry after a few seconds." True, but time is relative. A few seconds is a long time for a baby. And you have to admit you would begin to feel "cross" long before two hours had passed; in some cases an adult can begin to see red after only five or ten minutes of being treated with this level of contempt.)

It is also said of these poor babies that they "always want to be the centre of everyone's attention", which is a gross exaggeration. Babies have difficulty interacting with more than one person at a time; while one person is paying attention to him, he will take no notice of anybody else. He is content to be the focus of one person's attention.

Or they are labelled "selfish". A selfish person wants everything for himself at the expense of denying it to others. But the baby isn't denying anything to anyone; he is willing to respond, to exchange smiles and "gagas". In fact if anything he will lose out in the exchange, for if we aren't careful he will drool all over us, and it is very difficult for an adult to drool over a baby to the same extent. Far from being "selfish", the baby's intention is pure and selfless; a human interaction in which both parties come out winning.

Babies are said to be "play-acting to attract our attention", their tears aren't "real tears", as if the pain the child is showing wasn't genuine and he is just pretending to cry in order to "manipulate" us. Perhaps it is understandable for the mother and her friend to see it that way; one minute the baby is smiling and saying "gaga", they look away for a moment and the next thing they know he is howling pitifully. The change seems too abrupt; it is easy to suspect it is "false". But you, as an observer of children, have seen the look of genuine, deep distress on the little fellow's face; an anguished expression, which couldn't have been "play-acting" because the baby showed it precisely during the few seconds when no one was looking. A while back, I had the opportunity of seeing that expression in a scientific film made by a group of psychologists. A mother was instructed to sit opposite her child, and to smile at him and talk to him in a normal way for a couple of minutes. All of a sudden, she stopped talking or smiling or moving a muscle and remained completely still in front of the child for two minutes. One camera filmed the mother's face and the other the child's face and the two images were projected side by side on the screen. The baby's distress at the mother's lack of response was palpable, and it was also clear that no mother would have been able to tolerate the experiment for more than a couple of minutes. (Children of mothers who suffer from severe depression and are unresponsive towards their newborn babies can develop psychological problems.)[30]

So, why do babies behave in this way – if not out of jealousy, selfishness, to get attention, or out of sheer wickedness? Man is a social animal. He lives in groups. A baby's relationship with his mother is all-important, but his relationship with any other human is also crucial. He comes into the world programmed to "appeal" to the other members of the tribe, thus avoiding any aggression. He comes into the world programmed to "attract attention" from the other members of the tribe, thus obtaining their protection in case of danger. That is why, long before he can walk or talk, he is able to "interact" in a pleasant way with others. That is why when others ignore him or "leave him out" he finds it dangerous and distressing.

So, does this mean we must spend the whole day saying "coochie coochie coo" to ours and the neighbour's baby? Of course not. Firstly, it would be impossible: we have other children, other duties, other needs, and we can't give our undivided attention to one child. Secondly, our baby won't be "irreversibly traumatised" because we stop paying attention to him from time to time and he gets upset (although he would probably be affected in the long term if we paid him very little attention or ignored him completely). What I am trying to say is this:

1. We should lavish as much attention on our children as we can. It will never be too much. No child has ever been "psychologically traumatised" by an excess of smiles or from people saying "coochie coo" to them too many times.
2. When our baby cries or "throws a tantrum" in order to get our attention, we shouldn't think it is because he is naughty or capricious, but because he needs us and loves us.
3. An occasional smile, a caress, even a word spoken from a distance will help calm him at those times when we can't offer him our undivided attention. It will always be more preferable than following the tired advice, "He's just trying it on; let him cry, he'll soon get tired of it."

As the child grows older, he finds it easier and easier to tolerate being separated from his mother and being ignored by adults. He also develops more efficient ways of getting attention. When a stranger stops to speak to her mother, a little girl of two, five or seven has various options. She may:

- Tug at her mother's or her mother's friend's clothes.
- Show one or the other a treasure she has just discovered, such as a cigarette end or a snail's shell.
- Barge into the conversation with a more or less pertinent remark.
- Start asking, "Why?"
- Pick up slugs, kick up dust or stones, splash about in puddles or any number of things that will elicit an instant response from her mother.

What do all these actions have in common? Yes, you guessed right! They are all prohibited. They are all considered bad manners. They all risk making a mother angry and irritated instead of getting her attention. And this will cause the child to make even more of a "nuisance" of herself. Looked at in this context, these responses would appear to be non-adaptive, but only because environmental circumstances have changed. It is only in relatively recent periods (recent in evolutionary terms; a few centuries ago, say) that social expectations about what constitutes "good manners" have evolved. Doubtless 10,000 years ago, no one would have said: "It's rude to interrupt adults when they are talking", or "Children should be seen and not heard." Ten thousand years ago, there were hardly any conversations to interrupt, and no one cared whether a child's grubby hands tugged at or soiled their clothes. There were no jugs or glasses for them break, no homework for them not to do, no tables for them not to clear, no basins for them not to wash their hands in; nor was it possible to bother dad while he was watching the match. Most of the reasons why we shout at our children didn't exist yet. Like primates today, our ancestors probably shouted at their children mainly when they saw danger, when wolves were close by. When a child's parents shouted at him, it meant he must run towards them and be picked up;[11] running away from an angry mother was running towards danger, and it was the worst thing a child could do.

Our children have inherited this behaviour, and they often find themselves caught in a vicious circle. If we tell them off because they want attention, they demand more attention; if we scold them for interrupting, they interrupt more. They don't behave like that in order to disobey or irritate us, but because they can't help it. In fact, it isn't easy for children, the poor things.

Children the world over clamour for their parents' attention; however, the way in which this is interpreted can vary greatly. Langis quotes a story told by another expert, the head of the Family Education Centre.[2] During a course, presumably on family education, various adults were sitting on the floor and "a little girl of about two was amusing herself by getting up every two minutes and walking between us". The little girl's behaviour wasn't very respectful:

> [...] she thrust her hands in some people's faces and literally climbed onto others' shoulders. Most people there, the majority of them good parents, took no notice of her [...] until she walked past one member of the group, who gently took her arm, looked straight at her and said in a soft voice: "Run about as much as you like, walk between us if you like, but try not to tread on me, be more careful when you go past [...]." Half an hour later, guess whose lap the little girl was sitting on calmly? On that man's, and he was the only one treated to this privilege for the rest of the day.

For Langis this story shows that the man earned the little girl's respect by saying "no" to her. Children love to hear the word "no", they need to hear it, and parents should buy Mr Langis' book in order to learn how to say it properly.

My interpretation of the story is very different (you might argue that I can't interpret the scene because I wasn't there; however, I have seen many children involved in similar scenes, and the reader will decide which interpretation is closer to the truth). I don't think the adults in this group were "allowing" the child to "behave badly", i.e. they weren't being "lenient". On the contrary, they appeared to be "ignoring" her, not looking at her or speaking to her; they were playing the "ignore her, she'll soon grow tired of it" game, despite the little girl's continued efforts to get them to respond. I don't think the child was "amusing" herself by getting up every two minutes, I think she was bored to tears. At last, one of the adults touches the child, looks at her, engages with her in a friendly way. At that moment, a relationship is established between them, and he earns the privilege of having her sit on his lap. It was the friendly contact, the respectful look and the kindly voice, the fact of taking notice of her, which created the miracle. The actual words don't matter; if instead of saying, "try not to tread on me and be more careful…", the man had said to the little girl: "What's your name? Do you know how to draw? Go on, draw something for me on this bit of paper…", don't you think he would have won her affection just the same?

Dickens, a wonderful observer of children (and of human beings in general), has one of his characters tell a similar story in *Bleak House*:

On our way home, I so conciliated Peepy's affections by buying him a windmill and two flour-sacks that he would suffer nobody else to take off his hat and gloves and would sit nowhere at dinner but at my side.

Peepy is a small boy whose parents take no notice of him. The protagonist of the novel, a kind and very humble woman, attributes her success to the toy; but the reader knows that she has won his affection because of the attention she has given him, here and in previous chapters.

Why hasn't she started walking yet?

Polly absolutely refused to do any exploring in new worlds until she had made sure about getting back to the old one.
C.S. Lewis, THE MAGICIAN'S NEPHEW

But let us carry on watching children in the park. This time, our subject is a little girl of two. Her mother is sitting on a bench and she is playing in a sand pit. The little girl sits down, stands up, picks something up off the floor, wanders over to the swings, comes back, wanders over to the flower beds, comes back...

All these movements have one thing in common: they always begin and end with the mother. The little girl moves away from her in stages, stopping here and there to examine something interesting. When she reaches a certain distance, she decides to make her way back, and the return journey usually takes less time. That safety limit, the distance at which the girl turns around and goes back, increases with age and varies according to different factors (whether her surroundings are familiar or not, whether there are other people or animals close by, whether the space is clear or there are obstacles blocking her view of her mother). It also depends, of course, on how bold the little girl is. When she is near to her mother, she tends to walk longer and linger for a shorter period, but as she gets further away, she goes shorter distances and lingers longer. And when she decides to go back, she begins at a brisk pace then slows down the closer she gets to her mother. Sometimes she ends her expedition in her mother's arms or touching her, sometimes at a distance. After a while, the little girl goes off exploring again.

According to Bowlby, the mother is the "secure base"[31] from which the child carries out his explorations. Bowlby compares this to a group of soldiers making a foray into enemy territory. So long as they are able to communicate with the base, and know they can retreat if they are in danger, they are able to advance fearlessly. But if that communication is cut off, if the base is destroyed or retreat becomes impossible, the patrol becomes demoralised, and they cease being brave explorers and turn into fearful, lost creatures.

There is a two-way safety system: the mother and her little girl both maintain this contact, continually looking at one another and occasionally saying something. It is fascinating to watch, as precise as a symphony, although unrehearsed. The little girl can try a variety of methods to get her mother's attention, "Look what I'm doing", "Look what I found"; she will become more insistent if her mother doesn't look at her, or if she is busy doing something else. In the same way, if the little girl appears particularly absent-minded, the mother will try to catch her attention, if possible without alarming her ("Bye bye, Sonia", "Look, a pretty dog". . .). When the little girl reaches a certain distance, she will spontaneously turn back. If the mother thinks she is straying too far, she may tell her to come back (which doesn't usually do much good), or, more cleverly, she will try to attract her attention again ("Come and see this beautiful butterfly"). Or, if the latter fails, the mother will go over to her daughter. Unless there is a real danger, she probably won't go right up to her, but will stay at a "secure" distance. This, of course, allows the little girl to move further away because her secure base is closer to her. In some cases, when the child's safety limit is further than the mother's – for example if the child feels safe thirty yards away but the mother starts getting anxious at twenty – a rather comical pursuit can ensue. Some mothers think: "The little scamp, she charges off without looking back; if I hadn't gone after her, she would have got lost"; but in the majority of cases, the child would never have moved that far away had the mother not gone after her. Of course the child isn't wilfully making us chase her. When she goes further away because we are moving towards her, she isn't "trying it on", she is showing us she feels secure.

The little girl will automatically turn back at a certain distance, or after a certain time; but other factors may precipitate her return. One is a potential threat, such as the appearance of a dog or a stranger. Another is the feeling that her mother is no longer watching out for her; the arrival of a friend who begins talking to her will usually cause the girl to turn around and demand her attention. Here again, it would be mistaken to speak of "jealousy"; simply that a basic sense of caution tells her not to wander too far while her mother is talking and not paying attention.

Sooner or later it is time to go home. The mother calls her daughter, who more often than not refuses to come. Then she gets up and calls out to her again. This time, when the little girl sees her mother is getting ready to leave, she will probably go towards her. The mother now begins to walk away slowly, expecting the little girl to follow her. But she doesn't. She may sit down on the ground and begin to cry. She may run to her mother, stand in front of her, put her arms in the air and cry, "Carry!" between sobs. She may even try to clasp her knees to stop her mother from moving forward.

A scene follows, which we have all experienced or observed dozens of times. The mother entreats, shouts, commands, threatens, drags the child: "Walk, I told you!" "You've got two lovely little legs, perfect for walking." "No, I'm not carrying you, you're too heavy." "A big girl like you wanting to be carried." "You get on my nerves…" When two of you are struggling with the child, this can easily cause a mild disagreement: "Poor little thing, she must be exhausted…" "Tired, my eye! She's been leaping about all over the place. She's just trying it on!"

In some cases, the child attempts to follow the mother, but stops several times, lags behind or wanders off, and the mother, who is becoming more and more annoyed, keeps having to go back to fetch her.

Some mothers finally pick their child up and carry her (some almost immediately and tenderly, others only after a long struggle, exasperated, and roughly); others take the child by the hand and literally drag her away. The first are said to be spoiling their child, giving in to her whims, allowing themselves to be manipulated; the second to be training their child, to have learned when to say "no" or how to "set boundaries", to be "showing her who is in charge".

The children in the first group will calm down instantly, or after a brief cry, and within minutes you will see them being happily carried, as though nothing had happened; the others will be dragged kicking and screaming, and their mothers may accuse them loudly of "making a spectacle of themselves again" (as if the child were alone in creating the spectacle).

If we were able to see both groups of children (those who were "spoilt" and those who were "trained") aged five or six, we would discover that all of them are able to walk behind or beside their mothers without protesting, and none of them demand to be carried. If the child was repeatedly dragged, the conclusion will be that this was an efficient method of "training children to walk on their own", and their parents will be praised for their tireless resolve, for refusing to be manipulated by their child, and succeeding in quashing her initial signs of rebellion. And what of the parents who carried their child time after time? Will anyone apologise to them? Will anyone say: "You were right, you didn't spoil her, she is perfectly able to walk on her own." Of course not! Not only have those who warned, "You'll still be carrying her when she's old enough to leave home", not changed their minds, they have gone on to offer the fruits of their wisdom to other less experienced parents. They will never acknowledge their mistake, at most they will maintain a dignified silence, or possibly even try flagrantly to wriggle out of it: "Just as well she worked it out for herself or you'd still be carrying her."

For many, all the evidence points to the child's guilt: how loudly she cries, how well she was walking until moments before, how quickly she gets over it when she is picked up...; there is no doubt that this was pure "play-acting". The experts, however, interpret it in a very different way. Bowlby[11] examined the studies carried out by Anderson in England and by Rheingold and Keene in the United States. Anderson studied a group of children aged between fifteen months and two and a half years old and concluded that the abovementioned behaviour was almost universal. His observations convinced him that children of, that age are simply incapable of following their mothers. Bowlby bases his defence on the exact same evidence as the accusers:

Anderson's evidence strongly suggests . . . that up to this age [three years] transport by mother is the arrangement for which man is adapted. This likelihood is supported by the alacrity with which children of this age accept the offer of transport, by the contented and efficient way in which they poise themselves to be carried, and also by the determined and often abrupt ways they have of demanding it.

When he describes the way a child places himself suddenly in front of his mother almost causing her to fall over, he remarks:

The fact that a child is not discouraged by this untoward result suggests that the manœuvre is an instinctive one and is elicited by his seeing his mother in movement.

As for Rheingold and Keene, they made a systematic observation of more than 500 children in streets and parks, and discovered that 89 percent of those carried or wheeled in a pushchair were under three years old (with an equal number under one year old, of one to two years and of two to three years old). However, only 8 percent of children who didn't walk were between three and four, and only 2 percent were between four and five. On the contrary, most children between the age of three and five held a parent's hand or clothes or the handle of a pram, and only those over the age of seven were in the habit of walking on their own. Conclusion: this is a process of development relating to age. Children under three can't follow their mothers, not even if they take her hand, unless for brief periods and very slowly. Those over three, however, can.

Although these studies cited by Bowlby were carried out more than forty years ago, apparently many experts still haven't heard about, or understood, their implications. The "refusal to walk" is still given as an example of one the biggest indications of disobedience and resistance. Langis[2] cites it as a prime example of the first of the "thirteen ways in which today's parents are enslaved":

> The child always cries so that he is carried, even though he is perfectly able to walk for quite a long time on his own without getting tired. He is being capricious.[2]

Later on, the same author sees this as a classic example of the strange activity exclusive to childhood of "pushing the boundaries" and finding the tiniest weakness in parents' armour:

> A little girl tugs at her mother's skirt and demands again and again to be carried. The mother, worn down by the child's insistence, orders the girl angrily to walk beside her. The girl continues to tug at her mother's skirt, and the mother repeats the command. Then, all of a sudden, the mother decides to pick her up. It has taken the child less than fifteen seconds to get her own way.

For Ferreros, this is one of the only cases when you should never pick up a child under two years old:

> If he refuses to walk and we are faced with a typical tantrum. […] In the long run, it is better to ignore his bad behaviour, and, without saying a word, take him firmly by the hand and make him walk, even if at first he resists.[32]

Of course, now I understand, how could we possibly be so stupid as to pick up a child who refuses to walk? It is more logical to make a child who wants to be picked up walk, and to pick up a child who is willing to walk; that way we will be sure of upsetting both of them, and of making a fine spectacle of ourselves. Why not go and wait for your teenage daughter at the school gates and pick her up in front of her friends? You can be sure she will be pleased. (It is advisable do a few workouts at the gym before trying this, unless you want to put your back out.)

The mistake these authors make (in common with many doctors, psychologists and parents) is in thinking of "walking" as a single activity: the child "is walking", and therefore she can and should walk in every situation.

But this isn't true. Walking involves a whole range of activities. No one would dispute that the 100 metre race and the marathon are two very different events, and no athlete would dream of training for both. Likewise, for a child to walk around her mother while she is sitting still, or to walk beside her are two completely different activities. In order to achieve the latter, it is not enough to move one leg after the other without falling over, I must also decide where I am, where mummy is, and the best way to get from one place to the other, while both places are continually moving!

There was a time when people thought children would never learn to walk unless they were taught. Dr Stirnimann instructed mothers how and at what age this education should begin, and he advocated special massages and exercises.[33] Perhaps, dear reader, you understand now why some grandmothers are shocked that we don't "teach our children to walk". In their day, such instruction was considered de rigueur; nowadays, however, nearly every mother and every paediatrician knows that walking isn't a process of learning but part of a child's development: if a child receives affection and attention, and isn't hindered by reins and swaddling, she will learn to walk at the appropriate age, at just over (or under) one year old. She doesn't need to be taught. Similarly, your child's development will also determine when she holds your hand without crying, or walks on her own. Your child will do these things when she is ready, at approximately three and seven years old respectively.

Expecting a child to walk in the street because you have seen her walking for a while in the park is like letting her drive on the motorway because she is good at bumper cars.

Of course, there is no overnight change. For a long period, the child will be able to walk, but only for a certain amount of time, or when she has a special desire to, or when she is in a good mood… The other day I saw a mother walk past my house with her son of about two. Judging from the time of day, she must have just picked him up from the nursery. She was eagerly encouraging him to walk: "Look, now we're going to take a tiny mouse step, that's right, veeery good!" (she took a tiny step). "And now a great big elephant step (she took an extra long step). "And now a kangaroo step" (she jumped). The child played along happily, but I couldn't help thinking: "If they live four blocks away, it will be dark by the time they get home!"

Many children show remarkable sensitivity at this stage of development: the same child who cries for her parents to carry her, will be perfectly able to walk with her grandparents, because she is aware that they are no longer strong or agile enough to carry her. Some children will accept to walk when they see their parents are laden with bags. It is not infrequent in such cases for a grandmother to say to her daughter: "You see? She tries it on with you, but I've taught her how to walk." The grandmother is taking the credit that rightfully belongs to the child, who has made a supreme effort to walk when it is still very difficult for her. And, bearing in mind how often the child receives reproaches or sarcastic comments ("So, you can walk now, can you, but with mummy you make a scene…?"), she doesn't do this out of a desire for reward or praise, but out of sheer goodness, because she has a moral conscience and wants to do good whenever possible.

Why is he jealous?

Adults are jealous of their sexual rivals, and children are jealous of their siblings. What are the parallels between these two situations, which make us respond to them in similar ways and give them the same name?

Jealousy isn't exclusive to humans. In those species, such as lions, where the male stays with the female and protects their young, he will usually see off possible rivals. The male who cares for his young passes on his genes more easily, provided his young are indeed his and share the same genes. Looking after another's young isn't very advantageous from an evolutionary point of view. The instinct to look after one's own young is passed on better when it is accompanied by the instinctive tendency to show jealousy.

The female doesn't usually have this kind of problem. She is in no doubt that her young are hers, and she couldn't care less what the male gets up to in his spare time. But the lengthy infancy of human offspring makes it desirable to be able to depend on the father's company. If your man begins to fool around with other women, you might find yourself alone one day with no one to help look after your children. In our species both men and women are jealous, and they don't like the person they love looking at others.

So why do young couples who have no children get jealous? Jealousy isn't a conscious rationalisation. You don't feel jealous because you think: "If my husband leaves me, I'll have difficulty making ends meet"; in the same way, you don't feel hungry because you think: "I need 1,800 calories to keep my metabolism going." Both jealousy and hunger are sensations that occur spontaneously from within and make us do things.

Jealousy between siblings works in a similar way: children need their parents' attention and care in order to survive. If the parents pay attention to one child at the expense of the other, the other child will suffer. This is why when a baby brother is born, the logical response of his older sibling is to do all he can to remind his parents: "Hey, don't forget me!", that is, to demand their attention. This isn't a conscious act; the three-year-old child doesn't think: "I must start wetting myself again, have tantrums and stammer so my parents take more notice of me." No, the fact is that over thousands of years, children who acted in this way were more likely to survive, and their genes have proliferated.

Jealous children show a curious mixture of behaviour. They act in a babyish way in order to evoke sympathy, yet they also like to act more grown up to show they are superior to their younger sibling. They treat their parents with a mixture of "needy" affection and hostility. They show an exaggerated affection, bordering on aggression, towards their sibling, like when they hold him so tight they nearly suffocate him. They sometimes try to hit him, or more frequently they make fun of him ("He can't talk properly, he goes poo-poo in his pants"); they may also throw tantrums and have fits of rage, insult and hit their own parents whose affection they are attempting to win. This behaviour may appear very strange to us, but deep down it is no different from that of a man who suspects his wife is interested in another man: one minute he cries and pleads, the next he tries to be a model husband by doing the dishes and showering his wife with gifts; one minute he is attentive and loving, the next he reproaches her, or makes a scene, or tries to belittle his rival; sometimes he may attack his rival or even his wife...

Why are we surprised by this behaviour in a child when we consider it normal in an adult?

Sometimes the older brother is described as having had his position "usurped". This assumes that the reason he is jealous is because he has lost the favouritism he enjoyed as an only child. Taken to an extreme, this way of thinking could mean that we should stop paying so much attention to our children so they won't notice the difference when a newborn comes along. This may sound crazy, and yet Skinner suggests something similar in

Walden Two.[34] Parents should show no more affection to their own child than to another:

> "Our goal is to have every adult member of Walden Two regard all our children as his own, and to have every child think of every adult as his parent."

The great advantage of having such little contact with their own parents is that, if they die, their orphaned child will suffer less:

> Think what this means to the child who has no mother or father! There is no occasion to envy companions who are not so deprived, because there is little or no practical difference.

However, the cause of jealousy isn't the memory of lost privilege. Younger siblings, who have never been only children and who have therefore never been able to become accustomed to being "the centre of undivided attention", also feel jealous of their older siblings. The fact of having been lavished with affection during the first years more likely diminishes than increases the first-born's feelings of jealousy, or rather it makes him more able to tolerate them.

The closer in age children are, the stronger the jealousy, because the older child still needs the same amount of attention (kisses, cuddles, constant company) as the newborn, and thus there is a greater rivalry. Jealousy between siblings is perfectly normal, and it is absurd (and often counter-productive) to try to deny, repress or eradicate it.

We can help a jealous child by showing him our unconditional love. He must be aware that he doesn't need to be jealous in order to get our attention, but he must also be aware that we still love him in spite of his being jealous. We can try to channel his jealousy into more positive expressions, to help him show how grown up and clever he is ("Tell mummy how you helped me give Pilar a bath. I'm so lucky to have little Juan to help me!"). But we cannot want or expect a child not to feel jealous. That would be unnatural.

Imagine if your husband came home one evening with a younger woman: "Darling, this is Laura, my second wife. I hope the two of you can be friends. As she's a newcomer and feels out of place, I'll have to spend a lot of time with her, I hope that as her elder you will behave properly and help more around the house. She'll be sleeping in my room so I can keep an eye on her, and you'll have a room of your own because you're a big girl now. Won't it be nice for you to have your own room? Ah, and of course you'll have to share your jewellery with her." Wouldn't you feel just a little jealous?

The Oedipus Complex

> *He was, to say the truth, one of those fathers*
> *who look on children as an unhappy consequence*
> *of their youthful pleasures [...] and looked*
> *on his children as his rivals.*
> Henry Fielding, JOSEPH ANDREWS

Laius, King of Thebes, consulted an oracle, which prophesied that the gods would punish him for his sins. If one day he begot a son, that son would kill him and marry his mother. For a while, Laius tried to avoid conceiving any children, but the only contraceptive method available at that time was an iron will. Unable to contain himself, he impregnated his wife Jocasta during a drunken spree. The cunning Laius did not wait around, and gave his baby son, Oedipus, to a shepherd who was to abandon him in the forest. The shepherd took pity on the boy, and spared him. Oedipus was eventually adopted by a childless couple, and lived to be a man. Unaware of his true origins, he killed his real father in a fight (which the father started – remember he was a bad man whom the gods wished to punish) and married his mother.

This tale gave Freud the name for his theory: the Oedipus complex is the desire all boys supposedly have to kill their father and marry their mother.

Yet this isn't the story the ancient Greek tragedy is telling us. Oedipus had no desire to kill his father or to marry his mother. He did so by accident, because he didn't know they were his parents. When he finally discovered the awful truth, he was so horrified he put out his own eyes, while his mother and wife took her own life.

If anything, the myth of Oedipus is about the exact opposite: the irrational fear some fathers have that their son will supplant them in his mother's affections – a fear that drove Laius to spurn and abandon his own son. He sowed the seeds of disdain and reaped hatred, when he could have sown the seeds of love and reaped respect. For the ancient Greeks, the moral of the story probably went something like this: "Try as you might, you cannot escape the punishment of the gods and you will meet your fate." For the modern reader who doesn't believe in those gods, the moral of the story isn't, "Abandon your son before he kills you", but rather the exact opposite: "Don't be so foolish as to abandon your son, or you'll make an enemy of someone who would have been your friend if you had treated him with love."

Do we fathers all suffer from this "Laius Complex"? I don't know how common paternal jealousy is, but it certainly exists. The father can feel excluded from such a close relationship (I've heard many women say: "You can meet the father of your child anywhere, but you carry your son inside you").

A father's jealousy can be twofold: he would like to be the child's mother, and he would like to be the mother's child – as if he were attempting to force his way between mother and son.

Some people suggest that mothers who are breastfeeding let their husband give the baby a bottle occasionally, to make him feel needed. It is a perfect way to upset the child and jeopardise his feeding. There are plenty of other opportunities for fathers to help look after their sons: he needs bathing, dressing, changing and taking out for a stroll; there is shopping, cooking, cleaning, washing and ironing to do.

Occasionally, an exhausted mother will tell me she is scarcely able to sleep because her son wakes her up with his crying several times a night:

"Sometimes I bring him into our bed so he can feed when he wants; it's the only way I can get any sleep. But, of course, his father says it won't do and he'll end up having to sleep in another bed."

"How old is your husband?"

"Thirty-two, why?"

"Isn't he old enough to be sleeping on his own? If he still needs to sleep with someone else at thirty-two, how does he expect a three-year-old boy to manage?"

Of course, I am only joking when I say that. The father needn't leave the bed, the three of them can sleep together. I am simply pointing out that a child's emotional needs are at least as important as those of an adult. Children are generous and understanding: if they can sleep with mum, they don't usually object to dad being in the bed. Therefore I am surprised to discover that Skinner[34] seriously suggests that fathers go to sleep in another room. And not necessarily to make way for their sons. No, both of them have to go:

> "Oh, the advisability of separate rooms for husband and wife, for example. We don't insist on it, but in the long run there's a more satisfactory relation when a single room isn't shared."

This is the situation. First the child is removed from the room and then the husband. Reflect, dear reader, and decide which side you are on. When someone suggests you put your child in a separate room, ask who will be the next to go.

Speaking of good old Oedipus, on a number of occasions, I

have heard people defend an even more curious theory: some doctors, and even some psychologists warn mothers that sleeping with their son "will give him an Oedipus Complex". This is a prime example of psychology-fiction. According to the schools of psychology that believe in the existence of the Oedipus Complex (and not all of them do, far from it), this complex is a phase of normal development. The mother can't bring it about through her actions, because it appears spontaneously, and that isn't a bad thing, because it's normal.

When will she become independent?

Independence is one of the big themes in modern parenting. We all want autonomous children! Children who get up and go to bed when they want, who only do their homework when they feel like it, who decide for themselves whether they go to school or not, who dress the way they want and eat what they like...

Goodness, no! Not that type of independence. We want our children to be independent, but to do exactly what we tell them. Or better still, we want them to guess what we are thinking and do what we want without us having to ask them; that way everyone would see what good parents we are, how much freedom we give them, and how we never tell them what to do. Many parents rebelled in their youth (or didn't and wished they had) against an overly strict upbringing. They promised themselves they would give their children more freedom. And now they are astonished to find that their children do what they want with that freedom. Of course they do, what did they expect?

In fact, what many parents mean when they say, "I want my child to be independent", is in fact: "I want him to sleep on his own without calling for me, to eat well and on his own, to play on his own quietly, not to bother me, and for him to be perfectly happy when I go out and leave him with someone else."

Yet it isn't reasonable to expect that of a child or an adult.

Humans are social animals, and consequently our autonomy doesn't consist of living alone on a desert island, but of living in a human group. We need others, and they need us. A human adult should be able to ask others for help in order to obtain his objectives, and to offer help to others when asked. We are interdependent rather than autonomous.

A beggar who asks for money is dependent; he depends on the goodwill of passers-by. An employee who receives a monthly wage could be thought of as dependent: because he would be unable to work without the company, his colleagues, bosses or subordinates; yet we consider him independent because he has a contract and a salary. He knows how much pay he is due, and he has the right to demand that amount.

If a child calls her dad and her dad goes to her, she is autonomous. If her dad doesn't go because he doesn't feel like it, the child is dependent on whether her dad feels like it or not. When you take notice of your child, you are teaching her to be independent. After a separation (an illness, the mother's job, starting nursery), the child becomes more dependent: she needs more attention, more physical contact, she doesn't want to be alone even for a moment. If she receives the contact she needs, she will end up overcoming her insecurities; if she is refused this contact, the problem will get worse and worse.

There is a world of difference between a child who stops calling her mother because she no longer needs her, and a child who stops calling because she knows that however much she calls, her mother will never come.

Your child is a good person

> *[...] indeed I don't know any use there would be in having sons at all, unless people could put confidence in them.*
> Charles Dickens, NICHOLAS NICKLEBY

Many experts, no doubt with the best intentions, speak to us of children's behavioural problems: problems with feeding, sleeping, jealousy, violence, selfishness... Everyone tells us about our children's problems, about how to detect, prevent or solve them, about how they "manipulate" us, or why we need to establish boundaries for them. No one reminds us that our children are good people.

And they are. They have to be, out of necessity. No animal species could survive if its individual members weren't born with the ability to acquire normal adult behaviour and the instinct to reproduce it. It is easy to teach a lion how to eat meat or a swallow to fly to Africa. What would be difficult, and require completely abnormal teaching methods, would be to bring up a vegetarian lion or a non-migratory swallow. The vast majority of newborns, if they are suitably brought up (i.e. with affection, respect and physical contact), will grow up to be normal children and, later on, normal adults. Human beings are social animals and therefore the ability to love and be loved, to respect and be respected, to help others and obtain the help of other members of the group, to understand and respect social norms (in short, to be a good person), are normal aspects of our personality. A good education, religion and laws provide us with other things; yet these aren't essential for us to become good people. Our ancestors were doubtless good people when they lived in caves, just as chickens are "good chickens" without any need for schools or policemen.

Let us take a look, then, at some of our children's good qualities.

Your child is selfless

Laura, who is three months old, is crying her eyes out. She has suckled, had a nappy change, she isn't cold, or hot, she hasn't been pricked by a safety pin. Her mother picks her up, sings her a few sweet words, and Laura immediately stops crying. She puts her back in her cot and she instantly starts crying again.

"She's not hungry or thirsty, there's nothing wrong with her," evil tongues will say, "What the devil does she want now?"

She wants her mother, she wants you, because she loves you. She doesn't love you because you feed her, dress her, keep her warm, or because of the toys you will buy her when she is older or the private school you will send her to, or the money you will leave her in your will. A child's love is pure, absolute, selfless.

Freud believed that children love their mother because she feeds them. This is the so-called secondary drive theory (the mother is secondary, milk is primary). Bowlby, in his theory of attachment, argues the exact opposite. He says the need of his mother is independent from, and probably more important than, the need to be fed.

Why don't you as a mother enjoy this wonderful feeling of being given unconditional love? Would you feel better if your daughter only called you when she was hungry, thirsty or cold, and ignored you completely once you had satisfied these needs? No one would deny food to a child who cries because she is hungry; no one would fail to bundle up a child who cries because she is cold. Would you refuse to pick up a child who cries because she needs your love?

Your child is generous

Not long ago a worried mother asked me when her eighteen-month-old daughter would stop being so selfish; when she would learn to share.

Why is learning to share such an obsession with so many parents and educators? What good does it do a child to learn about sharing? As adults, we share almost nothing.

An example: Isabel, who is not yet two, is playing in the park with her bucket and spade, and her ball, under her mother's watchful and loving eye. Naturally, because her hands are very small, she is only holding the spade while the bucket and ball are lying on the ground next to her. Another toddler of similar age comes over and sits down next to Isabel, and, without saying a word, grabs the ball. Isabel has paid no attention to the ball for nearly ten minutes, and at first she goes on calmly tapping the ground with her spade. Calmly? A keen observer will have noticed that the tapping is becoming more and more forceful, and Isabel is looking at the ball out of the corner of her eye. For his part, the newcomer seems perfectly aware he is treading on dangerous ground; he moves the ball away, waits for a response, and then moves it back. In case there is any misunderstanding, Isabel warns him: "S'mine!"; then feels the need to specify: "Ball's mine!" The intruder, who is apparently still unable to form three-word sentences (or perhaps he doesn't want to commit himself), simply repeats: "Ball, baaall, baw!" No doubt afraid these words amount to declaration of ownership, Isabel decides to reclaim outright possession of the little green ball. The intruder offers little resistance, but while she isn't looking manages to appropriate the bucket. Isabel plays contentedly for a few moments with her newly recovered ball, then suddenly looks concerned. What about her bucket! This is the limit!

And so it can go on half the afternoon. Isabel will readily allow the boy to play with one or other of her possessions, or she will tolerate it grudgingly or she won't tolerate it at all. She will occasionally offer the boy her spade in exchange for her bucket. There may be some tears and shouting on the part of both children; but, in any event, Isabel's new "friend" is likely to enjoy quite a lot of relatively peaceful play.

It is also very likely that both mothers will intervene. And now something happens that never ceases to amaze me: instead of fiercely defending her own child, each mother takes the other child's side. "Come on, Isabel, let the little boy play with your spade." "Come on, Pedro, give the little girl her spade back." At best, this will go no further than a few gentle exhortations; however, it is not unusual for both mothers to vie with each other zealously in the generosity stakes (how easy it is to be generous with someone else's spade!) "That's enough, Isabel, if you insist on behaving like that, mummy will get angry!" "Pedro, apologise this instant or we're leaving!" "Don't worry, it's all right if he plays with the spade! My little girl is so selfish…" "Well, my boy's a little devil! I have to watch him all the time, he's always annoying other children and snatching their things…" And so both children end up being told off, like tiny warring countries that might have reached a friendly agreement if the two superpowers hadn't become involved.

Scenes like these, repeated a thousand times over, sometimes make us think our children are selfish. We would share a plastic spade and a ball without a second's hesitation. But are we really more generous than they, or is it simply that we don't care about those things?

It is necessary to put things into perspective. Imagine you are sitting on a park bench listening to some music. Next to you on the bench is your bag, on top of a folded newspaper. Just then, a stranger comes over, sits down and, without saying a word, begins reading your newspaper. After a while he puts the newspaper down (on the ground, without closing it), picks your bag up, opens it, rummages inside… Would you be capable of sharing? How long would it take you to tell the stranger off in no uncertain terms, or to grab your bag and run off? If you saw a policeman in the distance, wouldn't you signal to him? Imagine if he came over and said:

"That's enough, give the man your bag or I'll get angry. Sorry, sir, this woman doesn't know how to share… Do you like the mobile phone? Make a call, call whom ever you want… Be quiet woman, if you go on protesting, you'll see what's what!"

Our ability to share depends on three factors: what we lend, to whom and for how long. We may lend a book to a colleague for a few weeks, but we don't like a stranger picking up our newspaper without asking. We would only let a close friend or relative take our car out for a spin. A toddler has few possessions, and a bucket

and spade, or a ball, are as important to her as a bag, a computer or
a motorbike are to us. Time seems longer for a child and lending
a toy for a few minutes is as difficult for her as it would be for
her father to lend someone his car for a few days. And our child
also distinguishes between friends and acquaintances, though we
may not realise this. For example, which of the following two
sentences would Isabel's mother use to summarise the stories
mentioned above?

a. Isabel was playing in the sandpit with her little friend, and a
    stranger came along, picked up my newspaper and almost
    made off with my bag. I got such a shock!
b. A friend and I were playing catch with my bag, and a
    stranger came along and tried to make off with Isabel's ball.
    I got such a shock!

Of course, from an adult's point of view, any harmless,
defenceless, two-year-old child is a "little friend". But when you
are less than three foot tall, a two-year-old boy is a stranger, and
possibly even an "individual with dubious intentions".

A final example: Enrique, aged twenty-five, powerless to stop
his little boy Quique from crying, uses his car keys as a rattle.
Quique grabs the keys, fondles them, looks at them, fondles
them again. A little girl of six comes over and begins clowning
around: "What a pretty little boy. What's his name? How old
is he? (she is one of those precocious little girls). My cousin
Antonio is eight months old, he hasn't come today because he's
got earache". "Hello, Quique! That's a nice set of keys! Give
them to me! Look, you can have this ball instead." Enrique's
father is delighted with his son's new little friend, that is until
the little girl goes running off with his car keys, leaving the ball
in fair payment. How many fractions of a second do you think
it will take before Enrique goes after her to get the keys back?
Quique was willing to share but his father wasn't.

Our children are far more generous than we are.

Your child is equable

> *To cry forever you deserve, if you don't cry now.*
> Torquato Tasso, JERSUALEM DELIVERED

That is, he is inclined to be even-tempered. In simple terms, your child isn't a cry-baby.

What do you mean, he cries all day long? Toddlers, it is true, cry more often than adults, which is why we usually call children cry-babies.

What if they simply have more reasons to cry?

"But they cry for no reason", you will say. "They cry over nothing." Depending on their age, they will cry because the tower they have made out of building blocks falls down, or because we won't buy them an ice-cream, or because we take them to the doctor, or because they can't find our nipple straight away, or because we change their nappy, or because we dry their hair... No adult would cry over such things, of course.

And what makes you cry? Try an experiment: sit your one- or two-year-old child on your lap and tell him the most awful things you can think of: "You're going to be inspected by the Inland Revenue." "You've been fired from your job." "You're getting terrible wrinkles." "Your football team has been relegated to the second division. . ." He won't cry. The things that make adults and children cry are completely different.

Among the things that most frequently make small children cry are:

- Being separated from their mothers for two minutes.
- Trying to do something and not succeeding.
- Noticing something strange and not knowing what it is.
- Needing something and not knowing how to get it.

All of these are things that unfortunately can (and do) happen several times a day, whereas the things that make adults cry only happen once in a while. That is why we appear to be less prone to tears, but it isn't true. If our team were relegated numerous times a day, or we were fired every morning, or several of our closest friends died every day, we would also spend the whole day crying.

Your child is forgiving

Emilia and her son Oscar, who is six, have had a strong disagreement. To cut a long story short, Emilia wanted Oscar to have a shower while Oscar considered he was perfectly clean. Shouts, sobs, insults and threats ensued. An impartial witness would concede that most of the sobs came from one of the aggrieved parties and most of the insults and threats from the other.

This happened an hour ago. Which of the two do you think is now happy, busily carrying on with his things as though nothing had happened, and is even unusually cheerful and affectionate, and which of them is, on the contrary, probably still angry, resentful and grumbling? "Look, mum, see what I'm doing?" "No, mum isn't in the mood." "Can we go to the zoo on Sunday?" "Do you think you deserve to go? Do you think you've been a good boy?"

The boy's father, Arturo, comes home from work. Which of the following do you think he will hear?

a. "Mum got very angry this afternoon, you can't imagine what a scene she made. You have to talk to her."
b. "This child has been rude to me all afternoon, he refused to do what I asked. You have to talk to him."

Our children forgive us dozens of times a day. They do so sincerely, unreservedly, without resentment to the point of completely forgetting the offence. They get over their irritation much more quickly than we do.

Your child is fearless

Imagine you are queuing up at the bank when a group of armed men wearing masks burst in. If they tell you to lie on the floor, won't you lie down? If they tell you to be quiet, won't you be quiet? If they tell you not to move, won't you stay very still? Do you think a child of two would obey? Impossible. No amount of force, or threats, not even a pistol held to his head could make a two-year-old be quiet for half an hour, not ask to do a wee-wee or to stop crying in mid tantrum. Admire his courage and stop complaining about his "stubbornness".

Your child is diplomatic

Pedro and Antonio, two friends aged five, are playing in the park while their fathers sit on a bench, chatting. Then Luis, another child from their class, arrives with his mother. Luis is thrilled with the tricycle he has just been given for his birthday!

Three children, one tricycle. Who could be surprised if a conflict arises, when we have seen thousands perish for the sake of much more ugly things, like oil wells or diamond mines?

Pedro and Antonio, like all the dispossessed, are leftists, and think wealth should be redistributed among friends. Luis, like all the nouveau riche, is on the right and believes that what belongs to him belongs to him. There is a misunderstanding, followed by an altercation. Pedro (who is slightly older) grabs the tricycle, and Luis falls on his bottom and starts crying his eyes out.

That's done it! Luis's mother scolds him for not sharing his toys and for being a cry-baby. It has to be said she does this partly "to save face", when what she is really thinking is that the other boy started it and that her son's friends are a bit rough. Pedro's father is furious; he knows his son started the "fight" and probably also feels obliged to lay it on a bit thick in order to "save face". He scolds his son, shouts at him, bombards him with rhetorical questions, "Who do you think you are!", the sort that leave the boy completely powerless (because he knows that, if he doesn't reply, his father will insist: "Come on, tell me, do you think it's nice to push people over?"; but that, if he does say something, it will be worse: "Don't answer back!"). The ticking off has taken on such proportions that Luis has now stopped crying and is watching, more stunned than contented, as Pedro in turn begins to cry, and Antonio looks on aghast.

Finally, Antonio has an idea. He catches Luis's attention and makes him laugh with his best imitation of a character on the TV. Once the ice has been broken, he suggests a race, "to the fountain", Luis accepts. "Come on Pedro, last one there's a ninny!" And the three of them rush off.

What a clever manoeuvre! Antonio has come up with an elaborate strategy for defusing the situation, and Luis, even though he is the offended party, has immediately understood and has agreed in order to spare Pedro from his father's harangue. The three boys are now playing happily, the incident has been forgotten and the tricycle has been abandoned over by the parents, who are still disgruntled. Luis's mother may even exclaim: "Look, he's not even using the tricycle, I could have saved myself the bother of bringing it down!" Antonio's father is silent, but he is very proud of his boy.

Your child is honest

And how his honesty bothers us! We use offensive and condescending words to describe him each time he says what he thinks: "Why is that man black?" (Don't be offensive!) "I want chocolate!" (Don't be difficult!) "Look at that fat lady!" (Don't be rude!) "I don't like peas!" (Don't be fussy!) "Why do I have to wash? I'm not dirty" (Don't answer back!). When will they learn those useful adult qualities of dissembling, shrewdness and deceitfulness...? They will learn them when they realise that they will be spared many a ticking off by lying or by not speaking out.

The teacher has to leave the classroom for a moment and he asks seven-year-old Carlos as Top of the Class to take charge. The noble task of being left in charge consists of patrolling the desks, arms folded, and telling off anyone who is talking. One of the children stands up for no reason. Carlos, exercising his authority, tells him to sit down; the boy refuses. Carlos approaches the offending child, arms still crossed, with the vague intention of forcing him to sit down at his desk. They struggle, arms crossed, they start to giggle, and the whole class dissolves into laughter.

In the middle of this merriment, the teacher strides angrily into the classroom. Carlos tries to explain, but the teacher doesn't want explanations. He simply asks in a threatening voice:

"Do you think laughing is acceptable when you're in charge?"

"Yes", Carlos replies, and he receives a sharp smack.

The teacher repeats the question in a raised voice:

"Do you think laughing is acceptable when you're in charge?"

This time Carlos pauses before replying. He is in shock, paralysed with fear. He tries to understand what he has done to deserve this treatment, because he hasn't been hit for fooling around in class, but for answering a question. And he answered correctly: he told the truth. Clearly the teacher wants him to say "no". Can he say "no" and save himself? Carlos tries to explain it to himself, to find a reason to change his answer to "no". He can't. If the question had been, "Are you allowed to laugh when you're in charge?", he could have said "no" immediately (he didn't know it wasn't allowed, but he does now: the teacher's angry response has made it perfectly clear that it isn't allowed). However, the question was: "Do you think laughing is acceptable when you're in charge?" "Yes I do," Carlos says to himself, "that's what I think, it's the truth, and I can't give a different answer." He isn't trying to be a hero, he isn't trying to defy his teacher, he only wants to tell the truth, and, amid breathless sobs, he says once more, "Yes!"

The teacher gives him another even harder smack, and, eyes flashing, face bright red, he repeats the ill-fated question in an alarmingly intimidating tone:

"Do you think laughing is acceptable when you're in charge?"

How many smacks can a seven-year-old boy withstand? Carlos wavers, he thinks of saying "yes" and feels afraid. He concentrates, takes a deep breath, represses his sobs, and utters a pathetic sounding "no" before bursting into tears.

This scene occurred over forty years ago; and Carlos, as you will have guessed, was me. I don't remember the pain of being hit, or the humiliation. I remember my surprise, amazement, confusion and…, above all, my anger and impotence at having been forced to lie.

Your child is sociable

See how easily your child begins playing with any other child, regardless of class, race or what clothes the child is wearing. You will never hear your little boy or girl make racist remarks ("I'm fed up with those immigrants, they come over here in their boats and take over our slides").

Even if their parents aren't on speaking terms because of some past quarrel, children will speak to one another freely and without prejudice. Up until recently it wasn't uncommon for parents to try to control this sociability in children ("I don't like you playing with so-and-so, he isn't nice/isn't one of us/isn't suitable/is a bad influence").

Your child is understanding

I have just carried out a little experiment. I googled "children are cruel" in Spanish and found forty pages containing that sentence. Out of millions of Internet pages the sentence "children are affectionate" only appears on one, and "children are understanding" on none. (Update: I wrote the above at the end of 2002. Children are mentioned more and more on the Internet, but scarcely in more favourable terms. In April 2006, the sentence "children are cruel" appears on 330 pages; "children are affectionate" on twenty-four, "children are understanding" on five. The more obvious "children are good" appears 262 times, but this is of no use in my statistic because "good" often qualifies what follows. In two of the first ten entries on Google the whole sentence read: "Children are good soldiers because they are obedient, they don't question orders and they are easier to manipulate then adult soldiers." It makes you shudder.) Children are accused of bullying smaller children, of insulting people with disabilities and poking fun at them. But this type of behaviour is the exception, not the rule. It is true that, owing to their lack of social skills, children can ask embarrassing questions and stare at people who have a physical disability. Yet they are also capable of behaving perfectly naturally towards other children and accepting them as they are, regardless of what they look like.

I know a couple with several children, the eldest of whom is severely mentally handicapped. He is unable to walk or talk. For a while, he got into the bad habit when anyone (child or adult) went near him, of pulling their hair. His younger siblings understood perfectly that he wasn't responsible for his actions, and they were wonderfully tolerant. If they were racing around and one of them went too near his brother and had his hair grabbed, he would stay very still, visibly in pain, and call for an adult to come and extricate him. Naturally, if anyone else pulled their hair their response was appropriately robust.

Many researchers have confirmed that children younger than three normally show empathy, that is, concern for others' suffering. When a friend cries, they will often try to console him.

Bowlby[31] cites a scrupulous study monitoring the behaviour of twenty children younger than three years at a nursery school. Half of them had suffered physical abuse, the other half came from families with problems, but they hadn't suffered any abuse. The children who had been abused fought twice as much as the others, and they also displayed three types of behaviour not observed in the children who hadn't been mistreated: attacking an adult, attacking another child without provocation, apparently only to annoy them, and shouting at or hitting other children who cried, instead of consoling them.

Children who are brought up with love and respect are loving and respectful. Not always, of course, but most of the time. It is their natural disposition, because cooperating with other members of the group is as natural for human beings as walking or talking. In order to produce aggressive children, we must force them in some way, deflect them from the normal path. Children who are "brought up" by parents who shout at them will shout. Children who are "brought up" by parents who are violent towards them will be violent.

CHAPTER 3
Theories I do not share

In the first two chapters of this book I have attempted to explain the needs of young children and the reasons for their behaviour. However, as I explained at the beginning, I still fear some parents may read my book, and then read others that say the exact opposite, and subsequently apply a medley of everything, assuming that in the end we are all saying the same thing.

Consequently, in the following pages, I will examine some of the ideas with which I disagree.

Fascistic parenting

In her book *For Your Own Good: Roots of Violence in Child-rearing*, Alice Miller examines some of the recommendations of eighteenth- and nineteenth-century German pedagogues who belonged to a movement that has come to be known as "poisonous pedagogy".[35] Miller argues that the unstated final aim of such methods was to produce obedient subjects and that this "educational" system explains the triumph of Nazism in Germany among a population pre-disposed towards blindly obeying authority figures, regardless of how cruel, senseless or immoral their orders. Miller's book (in common with all her works) is a highly recommendable read. Below are a few passages from these experts of the past, which the reader can compare with current ones to see how we have progressed.

> It is impossible to reason with young children; thus, willfulness must be driven out in a methodical manner [...] But if parents are fortunate enough to drive out willfulness from the very beginning

by means of scolding and the rod, they will have obedient, docile, and good children whom they can later provide with a good education. (J. Sulzer, 1748, quoted by Miller.)

It is quite natural for the child's soul to want to have a will of its own, and things that are not done correctly in the first two years will be difficult to rectify thereafter. One of the advantages of these early years is that then force and compulsion can be used. Over the years, children forget everything that happened to them in early childhood. If their wills can be broken at this time, they will never remember afterwards that they had a will, and for this very reason the severity that is required will not have any serious consequences. (J. Sulzer, 1748, quoted by Miller.)

Another rule with very important consequences: Even the child's permissible desires should always be satisfied only if the child is in an amiable or at least calm mood but never while he is crying or behaving in an unruly fashion. [...] the child must not be given even the slightest impression that anything can be won by crying or by unruly behavior. [...] The training just described will give the child a substantial head-start in the art of waiting and will prepare him for another, more important one: the art of self-denial. (D.G.M Schreber, 1858, quoted by Miller.)

One of the vile products of a misguided philanthropy is the idea that, in order to obey gladly, the child has to understand the reasons why an order is given and that blind obedience offends human dignity. (L. Kellner, 1852, quoted by Miller.)

Even truly Christian pedagogy, which takes a person as he is, not as he should be, cannot in principle renounce every form of corporal chastisement, for it is exactly the proper punishment for certain kinds of delinquency: it humiliates and upsets the child, affirms the necessity of bowing to a higher order and at the same time reveals paternal love in all its vigor. (K.A. Schmid, 1887, quoted by Miller.)

These theories, born of absolutist and despotic regimes, bring the repressive model of the State into the heart of the family, transforming the father into policeman, judge and executioner (and the mother into a simple subordinate). Presenting the theory as "scientific fact" gives it a cloak of false respectability. Science is supposedly non-ideological, impartial and objective. Those who would never tolerate a repressive State currently accept a repressive pedagogy. In 1945, Doctors Koller and Willi, respectively director of the Basilea Women's Hospital, and head of the Zurich Infants Asylum, expressed their ideas in very similar terms. Their book[36] went into at least six editions in Switzerland in 1945:

> The infant psyche is so simple, so innocent, so easy to control that it scarcely presents any difficulties. It responds like clockwork to the prescribed feeding times, asks to be fed punctually, is content with the amount of milk it receives, remains calm between feeds and sleeps through the night. The mother feels proud and happy with her well-behaved child. [...] Some babies refuse to feed at the given time or demand more than the prescribed number of feeds, or they torment their mother every night by crying for hours. [...] If the mother responds to any of these displays of disquiet or ill humour, she will soon become a slave to the child and will be very unhappy. The sooner we correct her mistakes the better, because it will be much more difficult later on. It is a mistake to pick the baby up when he cries during the night or between feeds; it is equally erroneous to hold him or give him an extra feed. If, after a visit to the doctor, everything is normal, the mother should let the baby cry; sometimes he will conform to the prescribed regime after a few days, but it may take weeks. Simply place him alone in a room where his cries can be heard as little as possible. Older babies often try to captivate their mothers by crying. They scream frantically when she leaves the room or when anyone but her tries to feed them. We must be careful from the start not to take this screaming seriously.

Curiously, it is a Spanish author who most openly champions pedagogy as a method of political indoctrination: Rafael Ramos,

Head of Paediatrics in Barcelona following the Spanish Civil War (1936–39) and Franco's victory in 1939. In his work dating from 1941,[37] he doesn't try to hide his political sympathies:

And the true State is one that pursues the happiness of its subjects even though in order to do so it sometimes needs to impose itself by force, to be hard, rigorous.

Of course the best thing is if the subject is brought up to be obedient from the start so that the State needn't use force:

From the day he is born, the child must be aware at all times that he will be cared for by someone superior to him, someone who will not simply feed him and keep him warm, but will curb his instincts: his mother […].

a) The child should be placed in his cot from the moment he is born onwards, and only be brought to his mother's bed to breastfeed. If he cries, he must not be picked up or cradled, but he should be cleaned if he soils himself, fed at the proper time, and kept warm if he is cold […] or, if he cries simply out of the need to cry and not because there is something wrong, he should be calmly left to cry […]. If scientific evidence weren't enough, the documented experience of many mothers shows that a newborn will cry for the first ten, twelve or fifteen days. However, if a strict approach of not picking him up, or calming him or giving him a dummy is adhered to, once that period has elapsed, convinced of the uselessness of his protests, the intensity of the baby's cries will diminish […].

b) He should not be breastfed every time he cries, only when his feed is due in a methodical way […]. The mother will often complain of the demands of feeding her child punctually, but how trivial this is in comparison with the time and effort she would need to devote to him if, because of her neglect, he were to contract some illness or disorder!

c) Without giving in to his whims, when the child begins to understand (which, although he does not show it, is sooner than one might think), he must be made to see that this strict approach is for his own good.

Thus, an invaluable seed is planted in the child's consciousness, which his mother will gradually nourish. The child will understand that he is subject to the will of another, who looks after him, controls him, and from whom he receives punishment, if for no other reason than his own happiness. How easy it will be for this child, later to become a man, to obey a higher authority! However, if the man he becomes hasn't received that upbringing from a tender age, he will tolerate no opposition, defying his teacher, his boss, the police, the State that governs him...

Let us examine the main philosophical principles ranged against the affectionate bond between mother and child:

- The intrinsic badness of the newborn baby: a capricious being, who manipulates his carers and makes demands he doesn't need, simply in order to be difficult. He will only acquire the moral values of an adult by means of a thoroughly repressive education. This clashes strongly with the old Christian idea of the child as an innocent who cannot rationalise, and who has no need to go to confession before he reaches the age of seven because he is incapable of sinning.
- The child who cries "out of the need to cry". Crying is not recognised as a symptom of suffering, rather as a normal, harmless (when not wicked) activity of the child.
- The demand for the mother's self-sacrifice. Although the mother's right to rest is occasionally invoked in order to justify these strict parenting rules, a conflicting version is given here – one which is closer to the truth: the mother has a tendency to pick up her child and to respond to his crying, and in doing so she runs the risk of spoiling him through simple "neglect". Sticking to the rules and the timetable is

difficult, and the mother complains about it, but she must sacrifice herself to prevent her child from falling ill.
• It is for his own good. The strictest treatment is encouraged, not for the good of the mother but for that of her own child.

At the same time some of the most traditional methods are used to impose these ideas on mothers:

• Scientific authority (when in fact the opinions given are personal and lack any scientific basis).
• Threats and emotional blackmail: the child will fall ill if these rules aren't adhered to.

Ramos's work also clearly demonstrates the political implications of parenting: the child's absolute submission is only a preparation for the submission of the adult.

Unfortunately, such pedagogic theories didn't disappear along with the dictatorship that advocated them. Authors, who undoubtedly do not share Dr Ramos's political ideas, continue to share his ideas on parenting. Fifty years on, we come across the same idea of the manipulative, devious child:

If [the cause] is remedied and he continues crying, be patient and let him cry. When the child realises no one is paying him any attention, he will stop. Otherwise, even the youngest baby will soon become aware of his power and will repeat the scene, giving way disastrously to the beginning of a bad upbringing. *Babies are much cleverer than people think.* (Ramos, 1941.)[37]

[...] Juan is intelligent, very intelligent, and he won't bend to our will without a struggle. Besides asking for water, saying ouch..., ruses we have already discussed, he may vomit. Don't be alarmed, there is nothing wrong with him: children are easily able to make themselves vomit. (Estivill, 1995.)[15]

And the myth of the self-sacrificing mother, and imposing rules on parents by means of threats and emotional blackmail:

> Raising and educating a child naturally involves sacrifice and takes up much of a mother's time. And yet her child's health and happiness will soon compensate her more than enough. Not doing so, allowing herself to be softened by his blessed crying, is to mistreat the child and turn him into a miserable wretch. (Ramos, 1941)[37]

> My son goes to sleep after eleven at night because my husband doesn't get home until then, and he wants to see the boy. Are we doing the wrong thing?
> [*Answer.*] Enjoying your child without taking into account his biological needs is a somewhat selfish attitude [...]. Remember that between the ages of five and seven months you are above all trying to help your child get into the habit of sleeping properly, and if you don't it will affect his physical and mental health. (Estivill, 1995.)[15]

Orderliness

> *Plenty of amusement and fresh air, but all within*
> *reason and in a methodical orderly fashion.*
> Leopoldo Alas, Clarin, DON URBANO

The idea that children need orderly lives with fixed routines is nothing new:

> Food and drink, clothing, sleep, and indeed the child's entire little household must be orderly and must never be altered in the least to accommodate their willfulness or whims so that they may learn in earliest childhood to submit strictly to the rules of orderliness. [. . .] if children become accustomed to orderliness

at a very early age, they will suppose thereafter that this is completely natural because they no longer realize that it has been artfully instilled in them [Sulzer, 1748, quoted by Miller.][35]

Two centuries later, other experts continue to defend the same ideas, although with different arguments:

A baby's education begins on the very first day; we must immediately accustom him to the idea that someone is guiding him. We must from the outset observe a strict order of sleeping and feeding times, and we should never allow him to impose his will on us with tears. If we yield to him even once, it will be etched on the baby's memory, and he will instantly try to manipulate us. (Stirnimann, 1947.)[33]

During the first year of his life, the child evolves very fast; in order to facilitate his first steps, his parents and educators must channel their energies into helping him to acquire good habits. [...] At this early stage of his development, the child needs to organise his life around external markers that provide him with a rhythm and order that are consistent with the pattern of his biological development. (Ferrerós, 1999.)[32]

After 250 years, only the method of selling the product has changed. In the past, the real reasons were clearly explained: order is something artificial parents impose for their own convenience, deceiving their children into bending to their will. The main aim is to accustom children to being obedient, and to make them believe the orders received are in fact their own needs. Two hundred years later, Stirnimann expressed himself in the same terms. Today, we are more politically correct (which is the politically correct way of saying we are hypocrites), and we try to pass order off as a need that stems from the child's biological development, the primary aim being to help the child.

Is it not an amazing coincidence that, with complete

disrespect for the child, educators in the past decided to "artificially instill" an order that just happened to be the one children "need"? And, if a child's development is biological (that is, internal, originating from within the child), why the need for "external markers"?

Researchers and reliable studies have no doubt contributed to the importance we give to routines. Bowlby,[38] for example, cites a study carried out by Peck and Havighurst in an American town in the 1940s and 1950s. They closely followed a group of children over a period of several years in order to evaluate the development of their characters and how it was affected by family life. The children most popular with researchers and fellow pupils were "well-integrated, emotionally mature, and possessed firm, internalized moral principles". Their parents approved of them highly, trusted them and participated in their activities, and were lenient rather than strict. These children's parents had good relationships. And here we come to our subject: "Home routine is regular without being rigidly so."

However, take note: only four of the children in their study were described as mature and well-integrated, and one of these had a different kind of family: "a physically unkempt working-class home, in which little regularity or consistency was seen by the interviewer". What is going on here? It wasn't orderliness that produced these likeable, well-balanced teenagers, it was all the other things: the love, trust and contact. Orderliness happened to feature in three of the four families because it was a value appreciated by middle-class families of the period. They may as well have said: "The fathers of well-integrated children wear ties."

And yet a shambolic working-class family can also produce a very mature and well-balanced child if he is given love and respect.

On the subject of orderly lives, the myth of sleep routines deserves special attention. A mother described her anxieties to us in the following terms:

The paediatrician told us we have to begin to provide him with a routine, but we mustn't let him fall asleep in our arms, which is very difficult.

The child prefers being held to being given a routine, and this is also easier for his parents. Why complicate matters? According to the myth, the child must always be made to go to sleep in the same way or "he will never learn". But life isn't static. Think of the way your child begins to take solids. Sometimes he eats his purée with a spoon (either with his parents feeding him or him trying to hold the spoon himself). Or his food is chopped up and he eats with his fingers (and, after a few months, with a fork). You may hold a piece of banana or a tangerine segment for him while he sucks it, or he will hold it himself. Sometimes he will sit in his high chair, at other times on his father's lap, sometimes he will munch on a biscuit or a slice of bread while he is being pushed down the street in his stroller. He usually eats at home, but some days he will eat at one of his grandparents' houses, and depending which, there may or may not be a high chair, the utensils and the food will be different, and they will put a different bib on him or no bib at all, and one grandmother will try to "play with him to make him eat", while the other will leave him to his own devices. He may even occasionally eat at his nursery school. Despite this complete lack of predictable routines, all children end up eating.

There is no need to eat the same food every day and there is no need for a sleep routine. But if there were, then why not choose the one that makes both you and your child happy? Falling asleep in your arms, or breastfeeding, or with you singing him a lullaby, or letting him sleep in your bed can also be routines: all it takes is to do them every day.

Behaviourism and education

> *For these and other similar reasons, they are of the*
> *opinion that parents are the last people who should*
> *be responsible for their own children's education.*
> Jonathan Swift, GULLIVER'S TRAVELS

Behaviourism is one of the many psychological theories that proliferated during the last century. As a theory it doubtless has its strong points, and can be useful in treating some cases. My intention here is not to assess Behaviourism as a whole, only one particular way of applying the theory to the raising and education of children.

One of the fathers of Behaviourism was B.F. Skinner, a psychologist who put laboratory rats into special cages ("Skinner boxes"). The cage was equipped with a lever and a small hole. Each time the rat pressed the lever, food would come through the hole. The rats quickly learned to press the lever in order to obtain food, and they pressed it more and more. The food was a "reinforcer" and the method was known as "operant conditioning". If you disconnect the lever and food stops coming through the hole, the rat will press the lever frantically at first, but soon gets tired and stops pressing it after a few days. This is known as the "extinction" of reinforced behaviour by withholding the reinforcer. If you want the behaviour to be reversed more rapidly, you can use a negative reinforcer: each time the rat presses the lever, it receives an electric shock.

Armed with his boxes and with infinite patience, Skinner learned a great deal about the behaviour of caged rats. He never studied them in the wild. Even so, his stroke of genius was to conclude that these discoveries could be applied to human beings, and that any type of behaviour could be "moulded" if the right reinforcers were used. In 1948 he wrote a science fiction book called *Walden Two*. Walden Two is the name of a kind of utopian commune, whose inhabitants have voluntarily isolated themselves from the world in order to live according to the teachings of Behaviourism. Techniques of reinforcement and education form the basis of their society. In the novel, which is written in a didactic style, Castle, a rather foolish professor of philosophy poses continual questions to Frazier, the founder of the commune, to enable him to show off his knowledge.

In *Walden Two*, children are brought up with almost no human contact for the first year in tiny individual cubicles with big windows. These are kept in a room where no one even watches over them (at least not when the book's protagonists go there):

> Behind the windows we could see babies of various ages. None of them wore more than a diaper, and there were no bedclothes. In one cubicle, a small red newborn was asleep on its stomach. Some of the older babies were awake and playing with toys. Near the door a baby on all fours pressed its nose against the glass and smiled at us.[34]

In the novel, the person who cares for these babies enters the room, which they half-jokingly refer to as the "aquarium", only in order to show visitors round. Needless to say, the babies aren't breastfed because their mothers are a source of infection:

> "What about the parent?" said Castle at once. "Don't parents see their babies?"
>
> "Oh, yes, so long as they are in good health. Some parents work in the nursery. Others come around every day or so, for at least a few minutes. They take the baby out for some sunshine, or play with it in a play room."

These babies, who sleep, play, smile and see their parents for a few minutes nearly every day, never cry because they experience no discomfort: the humidity and the temperature of their cubicles are perfectly controlled, allowing them to be unencumbered by clothes. Frazier doesn't hesitate to add:

> When a baby graduates from our Lower Nursery it knows nothing of frustration, anxiety or fear. It never cries, except when sick.

These words would anger any reasonably intelligent person. To assert that children who have spent nearly their entire lives inside a glass cubicle have never experienced frustration or anxiety is like a bad joke. The things that most resemble Skinner's aquariums in real life are the premature baby wards in hospitals, with their rows of incubators. And the children in there certainly cry. One of the most important advances in caring for premature babies is the kangaroo method: taking them out of the incubator for as long as possible and placing them in their mothers' arms; it has been shown that babies gain more weight, are less prone to illness and their heart and respiratory rates remain more stable (indicating that they are suffering less).[39]

However, in the novel the foolish Castle accepts, without question of course, that these poor neglected children are perfectly happy and even declares that they are spoiled:

> "But is it prepared for life?" said Castle. "Surely you can't continue to protect it from frustration or frightening situations forever?"
>
> "Of course not. But it can be prepared for them. We can build a tolerance for frustration by introducing obstacles gradually as the baby grows strong enough to handle them."

A few pages later, Frazier explains to us the educational methods used to teach children aged between one and six to tolerate frustration:

"How do you build up a tolerance to an annoying situation?" I said.

"Oh, for example, by having the children 'take' a more and more painful shock."

This astonishing declaration, the admission that he has subjected children to systematic torture, fails to elicit the slightest comment from any of the characters in the novel, not even from the two who are supposed not to believe in Frazier's theories. Later on he describes another slightly less extreme "educational" technique:

Take this case. A group of children arrive home after a long walk tired and hungry. They're expecting supper, they find, instead, that it's time for a lesson in self-control: they must stand for five minutes in front of steaming bowls of soup.

I have never heard any teacher, doctor or psychologist recommend administering electric shocks. However, I have heard dozens of suggestions which resemble the second technique: deliberately making a baby who is crying or a child who wants something wait; training him to "delay the gratification of his desires", to "put up with frustration", to "eke out his feeds". Some may think me extreme when I say that to me these methods are cruel and shameful. "You exaggerate", they will say, "making a child wait five minutes for his supper and torturing him with electric shocks aren't the same thing." Well, to Skinner they are; they are two perfectly interchangeable examples of the same technique.

Of course it won't do a child any harm to wait five minutes for his supper. He will naturally have to wait dozens, hundreds of times during his childhood. He will be hungry but dinner won't be ready yet. Or he will sit down at the table and be told to get up to wash his hands. He will want to watch a programme on TV, and he will have to wait for it to begin. He will have to wait for Christmas Day to open his presents, even though they are already hidden in his parent's wardrobe. A baby will wake up crying desperately, and his mother won't come for five minutes because she is asleep, in the shower or frying chips and they will burn if she leaves them. None of this will harm a child. Just as it won't do him any (permanent) harm if he accidentally receives an electric shock, or falls over when he is playing and bruises himself or scrapes his knee.

The real harm of all these "educational" techniques isn't the things in themselves, but the aim benind them. Accidentally touching a live wire or deliberately administering electric shocks to a child in order to teach him to tolerate frustration aren't the same thing. Any child would prefer to hurt himself playing than for his father to smack him, even if the smack hurt less. It isn't the same thing to say to oneself: "I must be patient because supper isn't ready yet", or "We can't eat until aunt Isabel gets here", as it is to think: "Supper is ready, but I can't eat yet because my parents want to make me wait." I wouldn't want any child of mine to remember me that way.

If a child is old enough to understand what is being done to him, he will presumably feel the same anger and humiliation any of us would feel under similar circumstances. Or perhaps Skinner is right: if a child has been subjected to such abuse from a young age, he will end up by submitting, by accepting that he has no rights, and is at the mercy of the desires and whims of others.

A baby, on the other hand, can't understand the reason for the delay; he will never know whether his mother was five minutes late because she was very busy or because she wanted to be. The baby, then, can't tell the difference, but the mother can. Acts of aggression can't be justified because the victim is oblivious to them. What is immoral is the act of deliberately causing frustration in a human being. If this evening the lights go out for ten minutes in your street, you'll never know whether there has been an actual power failure or whether the electricity company has decided to cut off the power for random intervals of ten minutes to teach citizens to tolerate frustration and to make do without electricity. You have no way of knowing, but you assume option number two is impossible. How could anyone do something like that to an adult, upset him on purpose in order to "educate him"? No, such things can only be done to children.

Walden Two is only a novel, yet it aspires to something more than that. On the cover of the Spanish edition is written:

> *Walden Two* isn't a diversion, the author isn't providing us with an entertainment. Skinner believes in his fictional world; *Walden Two* is recommended as complementary reading for students of Social Science in many American universities.[34]

He believes in his fictional world! He himself reaffirms this in the prologue he added in 1976, where he enthusiastically advocates the realisation of his ideas. Skinner never tried bringing up a child using his methods (it has been said that he applied it to his youngest daughter, but his older daughter strenuously denies this on the Skinner Foundation website).[40] The Israeli kibbutzim came closest to carrying out a practical application of his methods. Babies and children would sleep together, apart from their parents. The experiment failed, it was as troubling for the parents as it was for the children, and today in all kibbutzim children sleep with their parents until they reach adolescence.[41]

If Skinner had published a sham scientific article or carried out a sham experiment on non-existent subjects, his fraud would sooner or later have been discovered. His reputation would have gone up in smoke, he would have been hounded from his university and his books would have been forgotten. Instead, he invented a sham experiment using non-existent subjects, and instead of trying to pass it off as real, he published it as a science fiction novel. Ironically, many people accepted it as if it were real, or at least based on scientific evidence, and many thousands of psychologists and teachers have read his book and allowed these fantasies to permeate their beliefs and influence their lives.

The idea of systematically denying care and attention to children in order to increase their tolerance of frustration is currently widespread, as are many other ingenious uses of Behaviourist theories. But, in fact, these ideas were already old when Skinner tried to give them fresh scientific prestige:

> Now let us see how exercises can aid in the complete suppression of affect. [...] One such test is to go without certain things one loves; [...] Give them fine fruits and when they reach for them, put them to the test. Could you bring yourself to save this fruit until tomorrow? Could you make someone a present of it? [Schreber, 1858, quoted by Miller.][35]

Schreber, unlike Skinner, did educate his children using those methods. One of them, Daniel Paul Schreber, is considered "the most famous patient in psychology and psychoanalysis" (he was a patient of Freud, who wrote a book about his clinical case), and experts still argue over whether the way he was treated as a child influenced his subsequent mental illness.[42, 43] Another of Schreber's children, Daniel Gustav, shot himself at the age of thirty-eight.

In their wonderful book, *Why Are You Crying?*,[44] Cubells and Ricart give us a completely different theory about putting up with frustration:

> It is a common mistake to think that the best way for a child to learn to tolerate and overcome frustration is to confront him with it as soon as possible.

In their view it is parents, not children, who must learn to tolerate frustration. That is, we must understand that certain things frustrate our children, and they show this frustration by crying, shouting, having tantrums and even with blows and insults. We must be capable of putting up with these shows of anger, which are normal responses to frustration, without withdrawing our affection, without scolding or punishing them, without resorting to absurd reprisals.

A few myths regarding sleep

> *Some of the habits of our age will doubtless be*
> *considered barbaric by later generations –*
> *perhaps for insisting that small children and even*
> *infants sleep alone instead of with their parents.*
> Carl Sagan, THE DEMON-HAUNTED WORLD

Nightfall has always been a good time for storytelling; tales that send you to sleep and tales that keep you awake. Many tales are also told about sleep itself, and unfortunately some try to pass themselves off as fact.

Sleeping through the night

In the traditional version of the myth, children sleep eight or ten hours in a row; nowadays you will find even more outrageous versions in print:

A baby of six or at most seven months should be able to sleep on her own in a separate room in the dark, and to sleep through the night (for eleven or twelve hours in a row).[15]

Using a similar approach, Hollyer and Smith[45] claim that any child can and should sleep twelve hours in a row from the age of three months.

These experts don't tell us where they obtained this

information. We would like to think they didn't make it up, that the idea of normal children sleeping eleven or twelve hours (not eight or thirteen) from the age of six or three months (and not two or ten) came from somewhere.

After a lengthy search, I discovered a scientific study that may have given rise to this belief. It is a serious, well-constructed piece of research published in a prestigious medical journal in 1979. T.F. Anders[46] filmed all the night long two groups of children aged two and nine months, and he observed that 44 percent of the two-month-olds and 78 percent of the nine-month-olds slept through the night. He doesn't say whether they were breastfeeding, but, judging from the time and the place (the United States), it is probable that most of the two-month-olds and all the nine-month-olds were bottle-fed. All of the children slept alone in their cots.

It is easy to imagine that someone who read this study a while ago and hasn't looked at it since, or who only heard about it at second or third hand, might have ended up concluding that all six-month-old babies sleep through the night. After all, six months is "almost" the same as nine (maybe they read it upside down), and 78 percent is "almost" the same as 100 percent...

Well no, it isn't the same. There are still 22 percent of normal nine-month-old babies, bottle-fed alone in their cot, who don't sleep through the night.

However, let us read the study in more detail: it turns out Dr Anders's definition of "to sleep through the night" is the one common to literature on the subject in the English-speaking world: "The baby stays in her cot between midnight and five in the morning." There are two problems with this:

•   If the child wakes up but doesn't cry, or if she cries but doesn't get out of the cot (i.e. if her parents don't take her out, because she can't get out on her own), she is considered to have "slept through the night". In fact, the film shows that only 15 percent of the two-month-olds and 33 percent of the nine-month-olds slept continuously, without waking up, from midnight until five in the morning.

• If the baby wakes up at a quarter to twelve or at a quarter past five, she is also considered to have "slept through the night", even though her parents take her out of her cot and have to stay up with her from a quarter past five until half past six. Personally, if I have to get up at seven to go to work and my child is going to wake up once during the night, I don't see much difference between her waking up at four o'clock or at six o'clock, do you? What I would really like (I know it isn't the norm, and I have no right to demand it or expect it, but it would be nice), is not to be woken up at all during the night.

How many children actually slept from the moment they were put to bed until the moment they were taken out of their cots in the morning – Dr Estivill's famous eleven or twelve hours? The answer is we don't know, because the parents who took part in the study didn't leave their children in their cots for that long, they left them for an hour less: an average of ten and a half hours. Only 6 percent of the two-month-old babies and 16 percent of the nine-month-old babies slept for ten and a half hours solid. Eighty-four percent of these children, who sleep on their own in their own room and aren't breastfed, don't sleep what Dr Estivill considers the "normal" amount of time. As we saw in previous chapters, the percentage of babies who don't sleep "normally" would increase even more if they were breastfed and slept with their mothers.

Who defines what is normal? Firstly an arbitrary, absurd definition of "normal sleep" is established, which flies in the face of scientific knowledge, and is so stringent that only 15 percent of normal children comply with it. Then it is claimed that those children who don't fulfil the criteria suffer from "sleep disturbances", and, unless something is done, there will be "very harmful consequences":

> In babies and young children, a tendency to cry easily, fractiousness, bad moods, lack of concentration, dependency on their carer, possible growth problems. In school-age children, failure in their studies, insecurity, shyness, bad temper.[15]

Nor is there any mention of which scientific studies back up these threats. Yet threats are pivotal to the method, because if we told parents the simple truth, for example: "If your child wakes up several times during the night it's perfectly normal, and it won't do her any harm. But it exasperates you, doesn't it? So we're going to explain a simple method to prevent your child from being such a nuisance." If this is what we told parents, very few would be prepared to apply the "treatment". No, it is far better to make them think it is necessary for the good of their child.

Lastly, this 85 percent of parents are persuaded that, unless they read the book, their "abnormal" child won't be "cured":

> [...] stick to what you have read, don't do anything that hasn't been explained to you.[15]

With a caveat like that, the book's success is guaranteed.

The dangers of co-sleeping

> *And now I suggest you go to your room,*
> *compose yourself, and wait.*
> Franz Kafka, THE TRIAL

Many parents choose to have their child to sleep in their bed, some because it is more pleasant, others because it is more practical. Yet the pressure is enormous, and it ends up making them feel guilty, as Rosa explains:

> *I have a twelve-month-old baby, and for the past month it has been*

impossible to make her sleep the whole night in her own bed; she wakes up at midnight crying and the only way of calming her down is to bring her into our bed. As we both work, there's a point at which we prefer to have her sleep with us so we can get some rest, even though we know it's bad.

Actually, they aren't doing anything bad. They are doing the best for their daughter (the only thing that calms her) and the best for themselves (the only thing that allows them to get some rest). Who, then, is bothered by this decision they have taken of their own free will?

Parents are made to believe that sharing a bed with their child (co-sleeping) is bad for the child. They will crush him, they will turn him into an insomniac for the rest of his life or cause him some deep and mysterious psychological trauma. Is there any truth in this?

No random controlled trial has been carried out (whereby one group of pregnant women would be asked to practice co-sleeping with their child, and another to sleep apart from theirs, and a study would be made of the long-term effects). All the data, therefore, comes from studies of an inferior quality.

Co-sleeping doesn't cause insomnia

> *When a mother sleeps with her child,*
> *the child sleeps twice.*
> Miguel de Unamauno

Many observational studies see a link between co-sleeping and various sleep disturbances. For example, Curell and his colleagues[47] found that among the group that practise co-sleeping, more parents (17 percent vs. 5 percent) and more children (44 percent vs. 17 percent) experience bedtime as something unpleasant; the children sleep less (10.4 vs. 10.8

hours); proportionally they wake up more (89 percent vs. 51 percent); they take longer to go to sleep (25 vs. 17 minutes), they are older (20 vs. 16 months); and they are more likely to have a low socio-economic status (51 percent vs. 29 percent). The authors conclude that "co-sleeping has a harmful effect on children's sleep", but they forget to mention that it also causes ageing in children and poverty... I am joking. Of course co-sleeping doesn't cause poverty; that is only a statistical association, in fact there could even be an inverse causality, perhaps certain social groups traditionally practice co-sleeping ...

Good, in the same way, the most logical explanation for the association between sleep disturbances and co-sleeping isn't that co-sleeping causes sleep disturbances, but rather the opposite: in a society where co-sleeping is generally frowned upon, parents only resort to it when their child has a tendency to cry or wake up or take a long time to fall asleep, and other methods of making him go to sleep have failed.

How, then, do we explain, for example, that 44 percent of children who sleep with their parents find bedtime an unpleasant experience, as opposed to only 17 percent of those who sleep on their own? Are we to believe that children prefer to sleep on their own than with their parents? Did these children want to sleep on their own in their room, but were forced to sleep in their parents' bed? Isn't it more likely that the parents first tried to make their child sleep on his own, but when he cried and resisted they grudgingly and irritably let him sleep in their bed? ("You're such a nuisance, you'll be the death of me. Come on then, come into our bed if that's what you want!") Something like that has to happen for a child to find going into his parents' bed unpleasant.

Transcultural studies shed some light on this point. In America, co-sleeping is usually frowned upon among whites, but is common and considered acceptable among blacks. Dr Lozoff and her colleagues[48] studied four groups of American children between the ages of six and forty-eight months: lower-class whites, upper-class whites, lower-class blacks and upper-class blacks. A greater number of poor white children co-slept with their parents (23 percent) than rich white children (13 percent), but among blacks there was no difference (56 percent of poor black children and 57 percent of rich black children co-slept with their parents). Co-sleeping was associated with minor sleep disturbances among poor whites and rich blacks, but not in the other two groups. Only among poor whites was co-sleeping statistically associated with parents' perception that their child had a serious sleep disturbance; in the other groups the difference wasn't significant, and among poor blacks the difference actually favoured co-sleeping (the children who slept alone had more problems).

How is it possible to explain all of these differences? Perhaps poor whites reluctantly share their bed with their child because of a previous sleep disturbance or because they haven't enough rooms in the house, while the few rich whites who co-sleep with their child do so convinced they are acting for the best because this is what they have read in books. Perhaps, poor blacks traditionally practice co-sleeping, because they believe it is normal and therefore it causes no problems and they encounter none; whereas rich blacks, although they have kept up the tradition, have read books or heard paediatricians criticising co-sleeping, and they begin to feel guilty about what they are doing and end up having problems sleeping.

The comparison between Japan and America is even more spectacular. Japan is a highly industrialised society in which co-sleeping is considered desirable and normal. Children traditionally sleep in their parents' bed until the age of five, after which they usually go to sleep in a grandparents' bed (if there is one living at home) until they reach adolescence. This is a mark of respect towards the grandparents: it would be bad manners to leave them on their own. From a sample of middle-class Japanese families, Latz, Wolf and Lozoff [49] found that 59 percent of children aged between six and forty-eight months old slept with their mothers or both parents, and had done so all night every night since they were born; while only 15 percent of white Americans slept with their parents, and almost all of them only partially (that is, not every night or only part of the night).

Parents in both countries were asked whether their children made a fuss about going to sleep, woke up frequently (three or more times a week) and if they thought their child suffered from sleep disturbances. (We are talking about perceived problems. This depends not only on what children do but also on what their parents expect of them: faced with two children with the same sleep pattern, one set of parents may consider their child has a problem while the other thinks theirs is normal.) Among the group of Americans, co-sleeping with their children was associated with them not wanting to go to sleep, waking up frequently and sleep disturbances. In contrast, the Japanese children who co-slept with their parents didn't have more "problems" going to sleep or put up any resistance, but they did wake up more frequently (since the parents supplied this information, the association could simply mean that parents who sleep apart from their children don't always realise when they wake up).

There may not appear to be much difference: in both countries children who sleep on their own sleep "better" than those who sleep with their parents. But now comes the really exciting part. The Japanese children who slept with their parents woke up in the middle of the night almost as infrequently (30 percent) as the American children who slept on their own. The American children who slept in their parents' bed woke up much more frequently (67 percent), while the Japanese children who slept on their own woke up very little (4 percent). Sleep where they will, Japanese children have far fewer problems, they put up less resistance and wake up less frequently than American children.

The authors of the study conclude that:

Resisting the intense desire of young children for close proximity with caregivers at night may set the stage for bedtime protest and persistent night waking in the United States. Other factors that may increase bedtime protest and night waking in US cosleeping children include intermittent and partial cosleeping, parental resort to cosleeping in reaction to a child's disturbed sleep, professional recommendations against the practice, and parental ambivalence about cosleeping.

And so the threat of serious consequences is completely spurious: not only does co-sleeping not produce insomnia, but it seems the attempt to force children to sleep on their own is the cause of sleep disturbances in the West. Could it be that our sleep experts are devoted to solving problems of their own making.

But why do children who sleep on their own sleep more in both countries, anyhow? Spontaneous selection has probably occurred, but the other way round this time: in America, where co-sleeping is frowned upon, only children who are unable to sleep any other way are allowed into their parents' bed; this is a selected group of children who don't sleep very well. In contrast, in Japan, where co-sleeping is the norm, only parents whose children sleep very soundly dare imitate what they have seen in films and put their children in separate rooms; this was a selected group of children who are heavy sleepers.

Spanish culture doesn't appear as obsessed with "sleep disturbances" as they are in America, although pressure has been mounting in recent years. Consequently, García and his colleagues[50] in a rural area of Catalonia, found that half of children aged between one and three woke up during the night, most of them more than twice. Many of them wanted company, water or food; most parents complied with these demands. But only half of families whose children woke up during the night considered their child "slept badly", and only one out of every five had consulted a doctor about it. Compare this tolerant and relaxed attitude of the majority of parents with the fearmongering of some experts: referring to "infant insomnia due to incorrect routines", Estivill[51] claims:

> There is nothing more unsettling to marital harmony..., the growing feeling of frustration..., self-blame is a frequent response...

In the past few decades co-sleeping appears to have become more widespread in Western countries, although it is difficult to know whether this increase is real or due to more people coming out of the closet about it. In America, 45 percent of children under seven months had co-slept with their parents at least once in the two weeks prior to the survey, and the percentage of those who habitually co-slept with their parents had increased from 5.5 percent to 12.8 percent between 1993 and 2000.[86]

Co-sleeping doesn't cause psychological problems

Like a young mother, watching over her first-born.
Julio Dinis, AN ENGLISH FAMILY

What is the basis of some people's claim that a child who sleeps in his parent's bed will end up in a lunatic asylum? As we explained earlier, an authoritative scientific study would require telling 100 pregnant mothers to co-sleep with their children and another 100 to put their children in a separate room, and then waiting twenty years to see which children have more psychological problems. No one has carried out such a study.

Cohort studies are less reliable. They require finding children who co-sleep with their parents and children who sleep on their own, and seeing what happens in a few years' time. As it is the parents who decide whether or not they co-sleep with their children, there can be a bias in the selection. For example, we saw that in America poor blacks co-sleep more with their children than rich whites; parents who are less educated, or who have financial or conjugal problems also co-sleep more with their children. And children who are ill or who have suffered an accident are also more likely to be admitted into the parental bed.[52] If when they are older these children behave differently, will this be due to co-sleeping or to social inequality or poverty or illness? Moreover, in a society in which co-sleeping is frowned upon, those who practise it may suffer from feelings of guilt and consequently treat their children with ambivalence or hostility. For all these reasons, we shouldn't be surprised if some cohort studies found that children who co-sleep with their parents suffer from psychological problems.

And yet, the only cohort study I came across that deals with this subject found no harmful effects in eighteen-year-olds who had co-slept with their parents as children: the relationships they enjoyed with their parents and others weren't worse, they didn't smoke or drink or take drugs more, they weren't more sexually active.[53]

Lastly, there is also a case control study; that is, one comparing children who have psychological problems with children who don't, to see which of them co-sleep more with their parents. The study was carried out by none other than a group of child psychiatrists at the United States Army Medical Center in Honolulu.[54]

The first surprising result is that 30 percent of children of military personnel (between the ages of two and thirteen, the average age being five) co-slept with their parents. And this figure increased to 50 percent when the father was on board ship. When their fathers were away, children under eight co-slept with their mother on average two or more nights a week; for children over eight, the average went down to 0.6 nights per week. There was no relation between the frequency of co-sleeping and the father's military rank.

The second surprising result is that the forty-seven children, who saw psychiatrists about various psychological problems, co-slept with their parents less than the thirty-seven children in the control group. The difference was particularly marked among boys over three: five out of six healthy children of that age group co-slept with their mother when their father was away, compared with only eight out of twenty-two of the children with psychological problems.

Co-sleeping doesn't cause sudden death

Two centuries ago when all children co-slept with their parents, some were found dead in the morning. It was thought their mothers had accidentally suffocated them; it was suspected some of them had been unwanted children deliberately murdered. In order to prevent these supposed accidents, or to stop mothers from being able to commit infanticide with impunity, doctors, and occasionally the law, prohibited children from co-sleeping with their parents.

To everyone's surprise, children continued to die in their sleep, despite being in cots where no one could crush them. Today we call this problem Sudden Infant Death Syndrome (SIDS). However, only a few decades ago, the term commonly used by parents and doctors was "cot death". Ninety percent of these deaths occur in the first six months, the rest between six months and a year.

The precise cause of SIDS is unknown, but there are several known factors that can increase or decrease the risk. Unfortunately, the risk can't be reduced to zero, and some children will die whatever their parents do. However, we can prevent many deaths by taking a few simple precautions, the most important of which are: always put a baby to sleep on its back (face down is the worst, but on the side also carries some risk); refrain from smoking during pregnancy and for the first few months after the baby is born (and, while we're at it, why not give up completely; this would benefit both parents and child); and never leave your child sleeping on his own in his room (it is best for the cot to be in the parents' room, at least for the first six months). The mattress must also be firm (i.e. of normal thickness; not a water bed or an inflatable bed); and avoid having any soft objects on or in the bed or cot that could smother the child, such as heavy eiderdowns, pillows, fluffy rugs (natural or synthetic) or furry toys. The baby mustn't be too warmly dressed (babies usually need slightly more clothing than adults, but don't put him in a thermal vest, two tops, a pair of flannel pyjamas and then cover him with a blanket and a duvet in a heated room). It seems breastfeeding also slightly diminishes the risk of sudden death.

And what about co-sleeping? Does it increase or decrease the risk, or does it have nothing to do with it?

Some data suggests that co-sleeping can reduce the risk, in certain circumstances at least. SIDS is very rare in Japan, where co-sleeping is most widespread, and it is also less frequent among Asian immigrant communities in England (who commonly practice co-sleeping) than among native English ones.[55] Furthermore, in laboratory studies, babies who sleep with their mothers sleep less deeply, which is thought to be a possible advantage.[56]

Various case control studies in New Zealand[57,58] and in England[59] found that, when the mother is a non-smoker, the risk of sudden death is exactly the same whether children co-sleep with their parents or sleep in a cot next to their bed. If the baby sleeps on its own in a separate room, the risk is five or ten times greater.[59,60]

Tobacco significantly increases the risk of SIDS. Smoking during pregnancy already increases this risk even if the mother then stops smoking (and even more if she carries on smoking).[61] No one should smoke in a house where there is a baby.

For reasons as yet unknown, the risks associated with

tobacco increases with co-sleeping. The British study,[59] probably the best designed to analyse this problem, found that smoking and sleeping separately increases the risk by five and smoking and co-sleeping increases it by twelve.

The ideal solution, then, is not to smoke at all. The mother who doesn't smoke, and hasn't smoked during pregnancy, can co-sleep with her child as often as she wants without any danger. Besides reducing the risk of SIDS, not smoking has many other health benefits for mother and child.

If the mother smokes or has smoked during pregnancy, it would be wise to refrain from sleeping with the baby for the first fourteen weeks (beyond this age, there is no longer an increased risk associated with co-sleeping even if the mother smokes). The baby can be breastfed then put to sleep in a cot, next to the parents' bed.

As we mentioned earlier, it is very dangerous to sleep with a baby on the sofa.

Other studies have produced slightly differing results. A study carried out in various European countries[87] likewise found that the incidence of SIDS increases dramatically when the mother smokes and co-sleeps with her child (the odds ratio is fourteen, which, somewhat simplified, translates as "a fourteen times greater risk"). However, even when the mother didn't smoke, co-sleeping was associated with a slightly higher risk of death (1.6 times greater), but only in the first eight weeks. I don't think this tiny increase should give any cause for concern: firstly, as I explained before, other reliable properly carried out studies have found no risk; secondly, other possible factors must be taken into consideration. In the same European study, if another occupant of the house who is not the mother smokes between half and one packet, the risk is 2.8 times greater (this increases to 8.8 times with one and a half packets or more). If the mother is aged between twenty-one and twenty-five, the risk is 2.44 times greater than if she is over thirty. The third child has a 2.29 times greater risk than the first-born. If the father is unemployed, the risk is 3.79 times greater. If the couple is in a civil partnership, the risk is 1.79 times greater . . . Obviously, a 1.6 greater risk, even if it were verified and re-verified as being causal (as opposed to a simple statistical association), is still very slight.

Although co-sleeping appears to be on the increase, in recent years the incidence of SIDS has decreased spectacularly in England[88] and America[89] as well as in other developed countries, largely due to the recommendation of putting children to sleep on their backs. The American Academy of Paediatrics[89] recommended in 2005 that babies sleep in the same room as their parents, although in their own cot. If the mother is a non-smoker then I consider this overly cautious, and in any case it would only be necessary for the first three months. The mother often falls asleep while she is breastfeeding, and having to stay awake in order to put the baby back in the cot can be exhausting.

It is curious the way new discoveries are accepted or rejected depending on whether or not they coincide with pre-existing beliefs. Many experts are quick to remind the mother of the alleged dangers of co-sleeping, while failing to explain that if she is a non-smoker the majority of studies have found no danger whatsoever. Yet very few remember that it is far more dangerous for a baby to sleep in a separate room during the first few months. And many insist, "The child is too old to sleep with his parents" (some after six months, others after a year, others after two years, depending on how tolerant they are), when in fact there is no evidence of any risk associated with co-sleeping after the baby reaches three months, even when the mother is a smoker.

Breastfeeding at night

We mustn't be persuaded by the infant's cries into breastfeeding him outside the proper time. If we begin feeding the child at night, he will become habituated and end up by demanding it.
Dr Fritz Stirnimann, 1947

It is usually said of babies: "After six months they don't need to breastfeed at night." The phrase is so meaninglessness as to be hard to refute. What does "they don't need" actually mean? That they won't die of hunger if they don't breastfeed during the night? That there are babies who don't breastfeed at night? That it is possible to prevent a particular child from breastfeeding at night? Well, by the same token, we could say: "Children don't need to go to school", "They don't need apples", "They don't need toys", "They don't need socks". No child has died (or even fallen seriously ill) from not going to school, not eating apples, not having toys or not wearing socks. There are millions of children who have never had such things. Any parent can deprive his child of school, apples, toys and socks if he wants. But who said that what is unnecessary should be prohibited? In the old days, prisoners in the dungeons were given bread and water, but no one checked to see whether they ate their bread and drank their water during the day or during the night.

There isn't much difference either between the words "children don't need to eat during the night" and "children don't need to eat during the day". Another expert could write a book explaining to beleaguered parents that children who eat during the day do so out of "learned bad habits" (naturally – they have learned to associate daylight with eating), and suggest a diet of four square meals a night, followed by eleven hours' fasting during the day. Dangerous? No more so during the day than during the night. Of course, parents who read both books and tried to use both methods at once, would have a very, very hungry child.

Let us leave aside the trivial question of whether children need to breastfeed at night or not, and concentrate on the really important thing: is breastfeeding at night bad for child and mother, or on the contrary is it good for them, and should it be recommended, or is it neither good nor bad, and would it be wisest to keep quiet and let the individual decide?

No one, to my knowledge, not even the most zealous advocates of babies fasting at night, has seriously tried to argue that breastfeeding at night is bad for the child: it doesn't cause cancer or baldness, or piles, or an "upset stomach" or "indigestion". In fact, it is widely acknowledged that during the first months babies can breastfeed at night. If feeding at night were dangerous for a child of ten months, wouldn't the danger be even greater for a child of only two months? The terrible dangers of breastfeeding at night would appear to be all in the mind: like the man-eating tiger that has tasted human blood, the child who has tasted milk at night will turn into a mother-eater.

I know of no evidence to back up such a theory. It wouldn't surprise me if the film *Gremlins* hadn't influenced the proponents of this argument – those sweet, adorable creatures, who, if fed after midnight, transform into homicidal monsters.

McKenna, an American anthropologist, studied[62] the connection between co-sleeping with the mother and the frequency of night feeds in a group of thirty-five children and their mothers, Americans of Latino origin (an ethnic group that considers co-sleeping a positive thing). Twenty of the children usually slept with their mothers every day, while the others slept on their own; all of them were exclusively breastfed. When the children were three or four months old, each mother spent two nights with her child in a laboratory. They were filmed with infrared cameras, while their vital signs were recorded in order to distinguish the different sleep phases. Regardless of what they did at home, in the laboratory each child slept one night with its mother and one night apart from her.

It was observed that the children breastfed more frequently and for longer periods when they slept with their mother than when they slept apart from her. That is to say, sleeping apart makes breastfeeding more difficult and therefore appears to diminish the number of feeds. Moreover, the babies who usually slept on their own at home breastfed less (on average 3.8 feeds the night they slept with their mother and 2.3 when they slept apart) than those who usually slept with their mothers before the experiment (4.7 and 3.3 feeds respectively). That is to say, habitually sleeping apart appeared to have a lasting effect on the children's behaviour, so that even when they were given the opportunity to sleep with their mothers they didn't manage to catch up completely.

For two weeks prior to the study, the mothers had noted down at home the number of feeds during the night. Interestingly, they fed less than in the laboratory: 2.4 feeds per night for those who slept with their mothers (4.7 in the laboratory), and 1.6 for those who slept apart (2.3 in the laboratory). This difference could be attributed to the children being nervous in an unfamiliar environment, but note that the difference is much more significant among those who sleep with their mothers (who, in theory you would expect to be less nervous). Perhaps what happened was that at home the mother didn't notice all the feeds because sometimes she was asleep, whereas in the laboratory, the implacable camera unerringly recorded every feed.

What is infantile insomnia?

When a small child takes a long time to fall asleep or wakes up several times during the night and calls her mother, they say she is suffering from "infantile insomnia caused by incorrect habits". In the Diagnostic and Statistical Manual of Mental Disorders (DSM-IV), a widely accepted international

classification, there is no illness with this name. However, there is one called "primary insomnia", the main diagnostic criteria of which are "difficulty initiating or maintaining sleep" and causing "clinically significant distress or impairment in social, occupational, or other important areas of functioning of the individual".

If my neighbour likes to go to sleep at ten o'clock, but I prefer to stay up reading until midnight, am I suffering from insomnia? Of course not, I would have insomnia if I went to bed at ten o'clock and couldn't get to sleep until midnight. Yet if a child prefers playing to going to sleep, he is said to be suffering from insomnia.

If my mattress were taken away from me and I were forced to sleep on the floor, it would be difficult for me to fall asleep. Would this mean I have insomnia? Of course not; give my mattress back and you will see how fast I fall asleep. If a child is separated from his mother and has difficulty falling asleep, is he suffering from insomnia? You will see how fast he falls asleep if you give him his mother back!

True insomnia, the kind some adults suffer from, is something completely different to this so-called "infantile insomnia" someone has dreamed up. I suppose there may be a child somewhere, who genuinely suffers from insomnia, but by and large we are speaking of children who either don't want to go to sleep, or who want to go to sleep but can't because we deprive them of the human contact they need in order to be able to sleep well. "Clinically significant distress" isn't caused by lack of sleep but by lack of human contact. We produce this distress when we are deceived by certain theories into denying our children the satisfaction of their basic needs.

Teaching children how to sleep

There are adults who don't know how to read or who have no

knowledge of geography because no one has taught them. But there is no such thing as a person who doesn't know how to sleep. Sleeping, eating, breathing or walking isn't learned behaviour. We are all born knowing how to sleep, eat and breathe, and we begin walking when we reach the appropriate age without anyone having to teach us. However, we can learn how to modify this instinctive behaviour in specific ways. We all know how to eat, but eating with chopsticks or a fork or a spoon has to be learned. We all know how to walk, but we have to learn how to dance. We all know how to breathe, but we have to learn how to play the flute. We all know how to sleep, but we have to learn how to do it in a particular way that is culturally acceptable (putting on pyjamas, getting into bed…). Doubtless our pre-human ancestors also knew how to sleep and didn't need teaching.

The greater the divide between the way we want our children to sleep and the way that comes naturally to them, the more we will need to teach them how to sleep. It is much easier to teach them to sleep in pyjamas or in a bed than it is to teach them to sleep without their mother. If they are with their mother, they will wear a nappy, pyjamas, anything you like. No child will make a scene in order to get out of wearing pyjamas or because they want to sleep outside on a bed of branches and leaves, which is probably the way our ancestors slept. There has never been any need to write a book about how to teach a child to wear pyjamas. Children aren't contrary; they will always play along and do what we say in matters they don't consider important. But when we try to make them sleep alone, we are asking something that goes completely against their deepest instincts, and they will put up quite a struggle.

A person who can't walk or breathe is ill. But a person who hasn't learned to dance or doesn't know how to play the flute isn't, and won't become ill from not knowing how to do these things. By the same token, if a child were actually unable to sleep, he would be ill (dangerously so, in fact, because a few days' total sleep deprivation would kill him). But a child who hasn't learned to sleep on his own, or with a doll, or in his cot, or when it suits his parents, isn't ill, and his inability to do these things won't make him ill.

Telling a mother that if her child doesn't sleep alone through the night, he is going to have problems sleeping when he is older is as cruel, absurd and mistaken as telling her that if he doesn't learn to play the flute he is going to have breathing problems when he is older.

Of course, those who advocate children sleeping on their own hold contradictory views on this question of learning. For some it appears children must be taught to sleep, an idea we have already refuted, while others acknowledge that the child already knows how to sleep, but must be taught to sleep in the proper way – that is, the way his parents want (provided his parents want him to sleep "on his own, in his room, through the night"; if the parents want something else, they no longer have any choice).

Lastly, the matter is sometimes explained the wrong way round. On this view, the norm, what all children come into this world equipped to do, would be: to sleep alone, to sleep through the night and not feed during the night. If they demand the presence of their parents to fall asleep, call them in the middle of the night or ask to be fed, it is because they have learned bad habits. This learning, it is argued, is a result of operant conditioning: the presence of their parents or of food acts as a positive reinforcer, increasing the frequency of reinforced behaviour (waking up, crying). Children must be "re-educated", they must forget the bad habits they have picked up, and return to "normal".

However, this theory has several weak points:

a. Why are there so few children who do what is "normal" and so many who "learn" what is abnormal? In many human societies, sleeping with parents or breastfeeding at night is considered normal and is widely practiced. Yet, even in our society, where such practices are considered abnormal and are strongly criticised, the majority of parents involuntarily

(!) "teach" their children bad habits. In the above-mentioned study by Curell,[47] 6 percent of children co-slept with their parents; but, of those who slept on their own, 21 percent fell asleep in "not recommended" places; 11 percent spent the night in an "not recommended" place; 64 percent of children and 73 percent of parents practised "not recommended" bedtime routines; 13 percent drank "abnormal" beverages during the night; 46 percent presented "disturbed" behaviour; and 51 percent woke up during the night. Altogether this makes 279 percent who were doing something wrong – that is, almost three things wrong per child. It makes one wonder whether a single child did everything right. If infantile insomnia really is an illness, then it is the worst epidemic in history, no one is healthy! Of course, among those who slept with their parents the number of sinners was even higher on all counts.

b. Why is what is "normal" (sleeping on their own) so easily forgotten, and what is "abnormal" (calling for their mother) so easily learned? According to this theory, parents, inadvertently and with no knowledge of pedagogy, are very quickly able to teach their children "bad habits"; by contrast, teaching them to sleep "normally" requires strict adherence to precise instructions ("Don't do anything that hasn't been explained to you"),[15] with clearly specified aims and methods, and complex charts with details of days and minutes. Thus, normal parents are excellent pedagogues, and in two days they effortlessly teach their children a very rare and difficult way of sleeping. Why not use the same methods for teaching your child ballet, atomic physics or Slavic languages? You will produce a genius! But wouldn't it be more logical if the exact opposite happened? Wouldn't it require a huge effort to prevent your child from behaving instinctively, and wouldn't he go back to that way of behaving at the first opportunity? Yes, and this is precisely what happens. It requires effort, method and consistency to make a child sleep alone, because it goes against his nature. But he will go back to calling his parents at the drop of a hat, because it is normal.

c.   The classic example of operant conditioning is the rat that receives food (the positive reinforcer) each time it presses a lever. According to those who believe in "incorrectly learned habits", waking up and calling for his parents is like pressing a lever, and the parents' subsequent appearance is the reinforcer. However, the first time the rat presses the lever, it does so without meaning to, because it doesn't know what the lever is for. Do you think a child wakes up and cries by accident the same way a rat scampering around its cage accidentally presses a lever? Isn't it rather that from the moment they are born, children have a strong inclination to call their mother? Calling the mother isn't learned, it is instinctive behaviour.

Moreover, the rat only presses the lever if food comes out and if it is hungry. If instead of food gold nuggets come out, the rat won't bother. Only what satisfies the rat's needs can act as a reinforcer. We work for money because we know money buys food; the rat has no understanding of anything that complex, and only works for food. Those who believe that the presence of the mother acts as a positive reinforcer are implicitly acknowledging that her presence is as necessary to the child as food is to the rat.

And so the brilliant suggestion, "Don't go to the child when he cries and he will stop crying", is the same as saying, "Don't give the rat food when it presses the lever and it will stop pressing the lever." The problem is if you stop giving the rat food, it will starve to death. And what about children, what happens to them if they are ignored?

Some parents don't want to let their child cry but they don't want to co-sleep either, or they would like to wean him off sleeping in their bed. If so, they may be interested to know there are ways of "teaching children to sleep" without letting them cry.[63] Of course, they aren't magic methods, and will require time and patience. However, remember you aren't teaching your child something he needs to know, but something you want him to know for your convenience. You aren't doing him a favour, you are asking a favour of him. If your child does you that favour, you should be grateful to him. And if he doesn't, well you will have to put up with it; the child is under no obligation.

A difficult habit to break

Man becomes accustomed to everything.
Almeida Garret, TRAVELS IN MY HOMELAND

In the abovementioned study[47], co-sleeping appears to occur more frequently with age: 3 percent of children under fifteen months sleep with their parents, as opposed to 9 percent of those between fifteen and thirty-six months. The authors draw the following conclusion:

> […] that co-sleeping is a habit and that changing or breaking a habit is difficult in the long term.

If co-sleeping were a habit or learned behaviour, this would indeed be the case: as with other habits or learned behaviours, the more frequently the behaviour is reinforced, the more it repeats itself and the harder it is to get rid of. It is easier for a little girl of four to forget to brush her teeth than it is for a forty-year-old woman. It is easier to give up smoking or drinking after a few months than after several years. Elderly people are usually very punctilious about their habits and any change upsets or confuses them. We remember perfectly from school how to add and multiply, because we do it all the time; but most adults would have great difficulty in working out the square root of a number, because we haven't done this since we were fifteen.

If after sleeping in his parents' bed for one night, a baby picks up this pernicious habit, after three months she will be a hardened criminal and after three years a hopeless sinner.

However, in medicine things aren't proven by reasoning but by research. In order to confirm that "breaking a habit is difficult in the long term", we have to observe these children over a long period of time and see whether they have given up the habit or not. Curell and his collaborators only studied children of up to three years, nothing is known about what happened after that. Other researchers,[64] who also readily brand co-sleeping a bad habit, obtained very different results in a rural area of Catalonia: 51 percent of children between five and twelve months co-slept with their parents; 28 percent of those between thirteen months and three years, and apparently 0 percent (or at least none are mentioned) of those between three and seven years. In America, Rosenfeld and his colleagues[65] also found that the frequency of co-sleeping decreased up to the age of ten.

That is to say, the "habit" is not only *not* difficult to break, but is broken spontaneously. Despite parents continuing to reinforce this behaviour (by letting their children sleep in their bed or going to them when they cry), this "learned behaviour" weakens and fades as children cry less and less during the night, and are more willing to sleep on their own. Your child will reach an age when she won't want to sleep in your bed for anything in the world. She will reach an age when she won't even want to share a room with her siblings (and when there are no more rooms in the house, this will create a conflict). These facts are incompatible with the theory of learned behaviour, and they prove that a child waking up in the night crying and wanting to be with her parents isn't a result of reinforced learning, but of instinctive behaviour appropriate to a certain age, which will disappear naturally at the right time.

Incidentally, if habits are so "difficult to break", why are the same people who want to prevent the habit of co-sleeping with the mother so keen to advocate other habits? For example:

> One of the two [parents] picks up one of your child's dolls
> and gives him a name, Pepe, let's say. He hands it to the child
> and says: "From now on, your friend Pepe will sleep with you
> always."[15]

Doesn't it strike you as odd that a child's friend should be a doll and not a human being? Because not only does Pepe have to be her friend, he has to be her best friend, because her other friends (her parents) are abandoning her when Pepe isn't. It couldn't be clearer: "He will sleep with you always." Won't relatives and neighbours start criticising? "She'll still have the doll when she leaves home." "She'll get married and take the doll to bed on her wedding night." Of course they won't – who would say such foolish things? We all know the child will sleep with her doll for a time, as long as she needs it, and then she will stop. She will sleep with it roughly the same amount of time she needs to sleep with her mother, for whom the doll is a sad, lifeless substitute. And yet, if you have been daring enough to ignore social prejudices and let your child sleep in your bed, I am sure you will have heard dozens of equally foolish remarks.

Leave him alone while he is still awake

Apparently, you are not allowed to let your child fall asleep in your arms or rock him in his cot, or sing him a lullaby or stay with him until he falls asleep. Advocates of this myth even go so far as to insist that if your child happens to fall asleep when he is not in his cot (whose child hasn't fallen asleep in the car on the way home from an outing?), you must wake him up so as to put him in his cot while he is awake.

This myth is justified by the belief that at the moment of falling asleep, the child experiences a kind of miraculous fixation on the things around him. If he wakes up during the night and doesn't see exactly what he saw when he fell asleep, he will panic and start crying:

> The child should associate sleep with a series of external objects that remain by his side throughout the night: the cot, his teddy bear etc.[15]

That is to say, calling for his mother at night is considered purely automatic, something the child has learned, and he will call her just because he saw her when he fell asleep. A teddy bear has the same effect, with the advantage that the bear can be there all night to calm the child, whereas the mother can't. (Why not? Because the mother minds having to put up with the child all night, while the bear doesn't. And what if the mother doesn't mind, what if she wants to be with her child? It makes no difference, she must do what the expert says and that is all there is to it.)

Curiously, among these "external elements" there is much mention of a mobile hanging from the ceiling or a poster on the wall. The minor detail that, when the child wakes up in the middle of the night, he is in complete darkness and therefore can't see anything (at which point, according to the theory, he ought to start crying until someone switches the light on), apparently does nothing to diminish the faith of believers. What about the baby who falls asleep on a summer afternoon when it is light and wakes up in the middle of the night? Or the baby who falls asleep to the murmur of voices or televisions, in his house or next-door, and wakes up in complete silence? Why does the disappearance of some external conditions appear not to bother the child in the slightest? Perhaps there are different categories, perhaps some elements are more important to him than others?

Let us try an experiment. Mothers, go to bed tonight with your one-year-old child and his doll. Tell your husband to tiptoe into the room at one o'clock in the morning, take the doll and go to sleep in a different bed. Tomorrow night do it the other way round: have your husband wake you at one o'clock and go out of the room the two of you, leaving your child on his own with the doll. Do you think your child will respond in the same way on both occasions? Of course not. When your husband takes the doll, the child won't make a sound. (Unless the doll is *the* doll, i.e. the doll some children take everywhere, what psychologists refer to as a transitional object. Such dolls are simply a mother substitute; children who are held a lot, and who sleep with their mothers don't usually have transitional objects because they don't need them.)

What the child calls for during the night isn't "the last thing he saw", because he isn't calling for a "thing", he is calling for a person. And not just any person. If your child falls asleep in the arms of a stranger, when he wakes up during the night, whom will he call, the stranger or his mother?

Is there any proof that children wake up more often if their parents are with them when they fall asleep? The only scientific studies carried out in order to confirm the truth of this statement are those of Adair and his colleagues in America. In the first study[66] they observed that one out of every three nine-month-old children went to sleep when one of his parents was present. During the week prior to the survey, the children who fell asleep unaccompanied woke up three times, and those who needed company in order to go to sleep woke up six times. The authors suggested a causal relationship (falling asleep in the company of a parent was what made them wake up), yet it is easy to imagine other possible explanations. For example, given that for years paediatricians and manuals on parenting have been advocating leaving children awake in their cots, especially in English-speaking countries, parents who don't follow such advice are likely to be raising their children differently in other areas. Or perhaps such parents feel obliged to stay with their children precisely because they sleep so little. Or perhaps they are parents who respond more to the needs of their children and therefore get up more often when they hear them crying. (In Adair's study "waking up in the night" meant the parents having to get up and go to the baby to calm him. The number of times the baby woke up without anyone noticing weren't counted.)

In a second study,[67] the same authors gave various parents of four-month-old children written instructions to leave their children awake in their cot, and even waking them up if they accidentally fell asleep. Nine months later they were asked to fill in the questionnaire from the first study. The children in that first study acted as a control group. The percentage of parents who remained with their children when they fell asleep had gone down from 33 percent to 21 percent. The average number of times the children woke up per week had gone down from 3.9 percent to 2.5, and the percentage of children who woke up seven or more times a week had gone down from 27 percent to 14 percent. Among the experimental group, the children who went to sleep unaccompanied only woke up 1.6 times per week, compared to six times per week for the children who fell asleep with a parent in the room. The authors conclude that their method is highly efficient. Yet they fail to explain how, given that it only changed 12 percent of parents' behaviour, it could be "so" efficient as to have made 13 percent more children go to sleep (that would be like saying, "This antibiotic is so good that of the twelve people who took it, thirteen got well").

It is also surprising that the children who go to sleep on their own in the first group wake up three times, and in the second group, 1.6 times, almost half as many times. Why such a significant difference if supposedly they are doing the same things? Either the number of times a child wakes up is so variable that the difference is random and therefore insignificant (in which case, of what value is the rest of the study?) or the parents are doing something they didn't do before. I was curious, so I wrote to the authors and asked to see the instruction sheet given to parents in the experimental group. It turns out that as well as recommending placing their child in the cot while he is still awake, it also recommended that if their child woke up in the night, parents "wait a few minutes" before going to him in case he went back to sleep on his own (Robin H. Adair, personal letter, 1992). We can assume that some parents followed both pieces of advice and others disregarded both. The parents who stayed with their child until he fell asleep went to him immediately if he woke up. The parents who left their child to fall asleep on his own, turned a deaf ear and didn't go to him if he cried. Given that only the occasions when the parents went to their child were counted as times when the child woke up, the above recommendation distorts the results, creating a false association between leaving the child awake in his cot and ignoring him.

Children, beds and sex

They say that a baby in the bedroom interferes with a couple's sex life. But that isn't true. When babies sleep they sleep so very deeply; and when the baby sleeps in his parents' bed it is possible, once he is asleep, to take him out and put him in his cot for a while. Of course, he may wake up suddenly, but that can also happen if he sleeps in a separate room, and if no one goes running to him, in two minutes he will be screaming his head off. Besides, the day is long and the house has many rooms. If you can't find a way of having sexual relations, don't blame it on your child.

An extreme version of this myth suggests mothers may put their baby in the bed as a barrier against their husbands:

> If there is tension between parents, then taking a child into their bed may help them avoid confrontation and sexual intimacy [...] instead of helping your child you are using them to avoid facing and solving your own problems.[17]

This type of comment seems to me insulting. Of course some married couples have problems, but why is this the first thing that occurs to some mean-spirited people when they see a child in his parents' bed? Why does no one say the opposite? ("If there is tension between mother and child, then taking a husband into their bed may help them avoid confrontation and the intimacy of breastfeeding [...] instead of helping your husband you are using him to avoid facing and solving your own problems.")

The comment is insulting, both to the mother (it accuses her of not loving her husband only because she loves her child) and to the father. If your husband is normal, the usual "I have a headache" is enough to "avoid sexual intimacy". If your husband were brutish enough not to accept "no" for an answer, would the presence of a mere baby put him off? And if this were the only thing stopping a wife from being violated by her own husband, what right have we to deprive her of her last, desperate defence?

The therapeutic cry

He eyed his good lady with looks of great satisfaction,
and begged, in an encouraging manner, that she
should cry her hardest: the exercise being looked upon,
by the faculty, as strongly conducive to health.
"It opens the lungs, washes the countenance, exercises the eyes, and
softens down the temper", said Mr. Bumble, "So cry away."
Charles Dickens, OLIVER TWIST

Crying is a very healthy activity, excellent for airing the lungs.
Stirnimann, EL NIÑO

And pneumologists still don't know this! Crying could turn out to be the best treatment for chronic bronchitis and asthma! But it is not my aim here to discuss crying and its effect on the lungs – a subject so clichéd that Dickens was already poking fun at it 100 years before Stirnimann brought it up again in all seriousness. No, I want to discuss a new, more insidious theory.

Doctor Aletha Solter recommends treating children with love and respect, holding them a lot, co-sleeping with them and breastfeeding them. Many mothers who think along these lines enjoy her books. Yet when it comes to the question of crying she makes a few claims that are more than debatable. Firstly, she attributes to tears a curious excretory function, as though they complemented the kidneys:[68]

> Studies have shown that people of all ages benefit from "a good cry" and that tears help to restore chemical balance to the body when subjected to stress.

And, of course, if crying is good for you, then we must let children cry.

> But if the baby continues to be upset or "petulant" after we have satisfied her primary needs, we should hold her in our arms lovingly and let her carry on crying.

I might agree with the above sentence if the child's needs really had been satisfied (and not just her primary needs). It is true that we don't always know what is the matter with a child, that we try everything and can't console her, and that at such times the best we can do is to hold her in our arms, give her our love and our company. The problem is Solter appears to be against consoling children when they cry:

> Our parents probably tried constantly to stop us crying when we were babies. Perhaps they gave us a dummy, or sweets, or they rocked us every time we cried, thinking this was what we needed.

Solter considers rocking, singing, breastfeeding on demand, distracting or tickling to be repressive tactics that prevent children from crying and are therefore harmful. Some mothers, convinced by this theory, stop consoling their children. And when, understandably, they cry even harder, Solter tries to convince mothers this is a good sign: at last their children are releasing the pent-up tears, suppressed by too much pampering.

No, I don't believe in this theory. It is the same old idea of letting the child cry based on a different theory as absurd as the one about airing the lungs. Solter denies the child the power to choose: if the mother thinks the child is hungry, she breastfeeds her because she needs feeding. But if she doesn't think she is hungry, then she decides the baby needs to cry. And who is she to decide whether the child is hungry or not, whether she needs to be fed or to cry? Anticipating that the mother has no objective reason on which to base her decision, Solter proposes a return to the fixed schedule: if the child cries off schedule, clearly, "it can't be" because she is hungry. The clock knows more about the baby's needs than the baby does! What Solter is suggesting is that we say to our children: "If I cradle you, cuddle you, breastfeed you or give you a dummy, you'll stop crying, but I'm not going to do those things because I want you to cry. I'll always be willing to hold you quietly in my arms, even if you are asking me for something else." This seems to me absurdly cruel.

I believe that children, like adults, cry in order to tell us something, in order to ask for our help. Normally, when we are alone, we cry or smile in silence. We cry or laugh out loud when we are with others, when someone is there to hear us. Children cry to make us do something, not so that we stand there and watch them. And if we feel better after a good cry, it isn't because we have eliminated any toxic substances, but because our crying has made others respond, because they have consoled and taken care of us.[5]

Family, limited company

For humans naturally desire
That which is most forbidden.
Torquato Tasso, JERUSALEM DELIVERED

Setting limits for children is another fashionable idea in the field of parenting. Whole books are devoted to this new science.[69] Naturally, limits are imposed for the good of the child:

> Limits are an aid, an important support, limiting the field of play within which the child can move freely in a safe and secure way.

Of course, it is important to set limits for children, because otherwise they would have no limits. Can you imagine what an awful situation?

A child with no limits would scratch all his friends' eyes out, would eat 200 sweets in five minutes, would throw himself off the balcony. A child with no limits would be a dreadful, shocking, repulsive thing, who…, who… How is it we have never seen one? What would a child with no limits be like?

A little girl with no limits

Marta feels very snug in bed, but her mum is calling her and she has to get up. Why can't she lie in for another half an hour?

Or better still, why go to school at all? She ought to be on holiday forever, go to the beach every day or ride her bicycle. Or better still, a horse. If she had a horse, she'd feed it sugar and carrots and ride away on her own and discover new countries. Well, not on her own, she'd go with Isabel, who is very nice…

Her mother's voice shatters her reverie. Yes, all right, I'm coming… What a bore, having to wash, the water's so cold. And the soap smells horrid. The soap at Isabel's house smells nice. I hate this dress. And these Acme® trainers are awful, all the other girls wear Cosme® trainers, but dad won't buy me new ones until mine are worn out...

Marta has long given up asking for more cocoa in her milk because her mum just doesn't understand that it has to be black. Round biscuits! The square ones are much nicer. Why should she brush her teeth after breakfast? But mum, my friends only brush theirs before bed. All right, I'm going... This toothpaste stings, why can't we have strawberry-flavoured toothpaste?

Marta has to carry her rucksack to school. She has to walk to school. Her mum doesn't want to take her by car because she says it isn't worth getting the car out to drive 200 yards. Marta stops in front of the toyshop window; she asks if she can have the electric train. "Try asking at Christmas", her mother yanks her arm. Marta stops to watch a dog peeing against a wall; another yank. She splashes in a puddle; another yank and a scolding.

School's a bore. You can't stand up when you want, you can't sit next to Isabel, you can't talk, you can't laugh, you have to look at the teacher, you have to listen to the teacher. Hand in your homework, open your book, take a clean sheet of paper, dictation, sit up straight, can't you see your pencil needs sharpening? Do the exercises on page 30, draw a cow, we'll finish page 42 tomorrow. "Now, Marta, recite your three times table... Since when does 3 times 6 equal 19? Let's see, can anyone tell Marta what 3 times 6 is?" "Isabel says she isn't your friend anymore because she saw you playing with Sonia." "Well you can tell Isabel she's stupid, and I can play with anyone I like." "Now, girls, what is so important it can't wait until class is over? Why don't you say it out loud so the rest of us can hear?"Oh no, not peas for lunch again! And that stupid Isabel doesn't want to sit next to me. Look at her talking to Ana, just to annoy me. Yuk, fish!

The return journey home couldn't be livelier. Her arm gets yanked in front of the bakery (No chocolate buns!), in front of the toyshop (No electric train!), in front of the computer store (No new games!), in front of the newspaper kiosk (No chewing gum!). "Marta, that's enough, you are really testing my nerves today!" (Yes, today, yesterday and every day).

"You have to change your shoes before you go out and play." "You have to do your homework before you can watch TV." "You have to stop watching TV this instant because supper's ready." "You have to help lay the table before sitting down." "I told you ten times to wash your hands. Look at the state of them!" "Oh no! I can't believe it! More peas! Mum, can I have a fried egg? Whaaat? Fish?"

"Is there any chocolate mousse?" "First you have to eat some fruit." "I don't want fruit." "Fruit is good for you." "I don't want any." "Eat a pear." "No, I don't like pears, are there any bananas?" "No, you can have a pear or an apple." "No, I want mousse." "Don't be rude to your mother, Marta." "Waah!"

"That's enough, here's your mousse, now be quiet!"

Stop right there! Dial 999! Did you see what happened there? Marta got her own way. All she had to do was shed a few tears, and her mother gave in immediately. Marta is the perfect example of the little girl who ALWAYS gets her own way. Totally spoilt. And all because her parents don't know how to set limits for her. They give her EVERYTHING she asks for. This little girl has serious behavioural problems:

> Children who see their every desire gratified are usually deeply dissatisfied, because in the end they can never have enough. Parents who endlessly spoil their children cause them to make increasing demands.[69]

No, don't be shocked. Nothing bad will happen to Marta because she "got her own way". On the contrary, the experience of getting their own way occasionally, seeing that sometimes they have control, that they can also do things, want things, achieve things, influence others, is probably necessary to the development of their personality. Because Marta, like all children, is constantly giving in and obeying, not dozens but hundreds of times a day.

When she demands mousse, Marta is learning to express clearly her point of view, and to demand respect; in a few years' time she will be able to do this without crying or shouting, and when she is grown up we will see that these qualities are positive. Her mother is showing Marta that she genuinely loves her, that she values her as a human being, and that she takes into account what she thinks and says. She is teaching Marta, by her example, to give in. If she wanted to do this properly, she could have given in in a more dignified way. Instead of shouting: "That's enough, here's your mousse, now be quiet!", she could have said, without raising her voice: "All right, if you prefer mousse, you can have mousse".

Should we always give in to our children, then? No, of course not. Not because it would spoil them, but because it would be impossible.

There is no such thing as a child without limits. Physical factors, which neither the child nor his parents can control already impose considerable limits. Your child can't fly, he doesn't always win when he plays with his friends, and he can't stop it from raining and spoiling a day at the beach.

There are times when you force him to do some things and forbid him from doing others for reasons that are more than justified (or at least you think they are, other parents may think differently): you have to go to school, you have to do your homework, you have to sit down and have supper, you have to wash your hands: you can't eat so many sweets, you've had enough ice-cream, we can't afford to go on holiday to Paris, the video game console is too expensive; I don't want you watching so much TV; you can't ride your bicycle into town, the roads are too busy; put your Meccano set away, we're going to see your grandparents; it's time for your bath, pick up your dirty clothes; don't touch the gas knobs; we can't have a dog in the flat...

If limits really are necessary for a child's happiness and for the development of his personality and character, then children everywhere, rich and poor, strictly brought up and "spoiled", have hundreds of opportunities every day to enjoy such limits.

Incidentally, why do we assume children need limits in order to be happy, that they enjoy them and are unhappy without them? Are children really so different, so alien, that their likes and dislikes are the exact opposite to ours? Limits usually have the opposite effect on adults: they make us miserable (unrequited love, holidays we can't afford, fat-free diets, cramped houses, our team losing a game…), whereas the things we achieve, and the aims we fulfil contribute to our happiness.

What truth can there be in the assertion that a lack of boundaries makes children unhappy?

Let us imagine, one Thursday afternoon, little Luis, with more or less dexterity, cutting some pictures out of an old magazine. Dad tells him he is doing it very well, and when mum gets home from work, he says to her, proudly, in front of the child: "Look how he's cut round the shapes and everything. It's amazing, and to think he's only two, what a clever boy." Emboldened, the following Saturday Luis gives a repeat performance; but, oh dear, shock, horror! Mum is shouting at him: "Look what you've done to the magazines, you wretched boy! I'm sick and tired of this child!", and dad joins in the scolding: "You've been very naughty, no TV for you this afternoon."

I suppose this is what people mean who claim children need clear, consistent limits and a predictable environment in order to be happy. The child can't be very happy, obviously, if what won him plaudits (or indifference) yesterday provokes shouts and punishments today.

But what makes the child unhappy, the inconsistency or the shouting? Because these parents could be more consistent in two very different ways:

- By praising him from now on each time he cuts out pictures from magazines.

- By shouting and punishing him from now on each time he cuts pictures out of magazines.

In both cases, the rule is clear and the result is predictable. According to certain theorists, both attitudes should make Luis equally happy. But we suspect the first option would make Luis 100 times happier.

If, on the other hand, we remove the shouts and punishments, then the inconsistencies don't seem all that bad. Sometimes Luis cuts out pictures and his parents cluck with pleasure. Other times Luis cuts out pictures and his parents don't say anything. Some afternoons, Luis cuts out pictures and his parents say, nicely, without shouting: "All right, that's enough cutting out for today", "Don't touch the scissors, you'll hurt yourself" or "Leave that magazine alone, you'll wreck it." Luis's parents' responses here are unpredictable, they range from very positive to mildly negative. Do you think this will cause Luis to be unhappy? I don't think so. I don't believe our children are that fragile or that we parents are that consistent. Most of us respond differently at different times, according to the mood we are in, the problems we have at the time or just by chance; and our inconsistency isn't limited to our treatment of our children, but includes many other aspects of our life. The ability to adapt limits to suit different situations is called flexibility, and flexibility is a quality we would do well to teach our children (by our example). The inability to keep to fixed limits is called human weakness, and understanding human weakness is a quality our children will also learn.

Furthermore, limits may be fixed, unchanging, clear, consistent and predictable, but our child may not know that. His age or ignorance may prevent him from appreciating all the nuances of a situation, and our logical, reasoned, rational responses may appear random and absurd to him. If it struck you as a little crazy the way Luis's parents changed their minds from one day to the next, rest assured, they are normal parents. But sometimes Luis cuts out pictures from used magazines, and other times from leaflets his mother collects. Sometimes he uses children's scissors, which are blunt and don't have a sharp point, and other times he picks up the sewing scissors, which could be the murder weapon in a movie. Sometimes he cuts out pictures during playtime, and other times he starts cutting out when it is time for his bath or his supper. Sometimes he does his cutting out in the corridor, and other times in the sitting room, covering the floor with confetti and digging the scissors into the Persian rug into the bargain. Aren't his parents right to respond in different ways? What difference does it make for a child whether limits can be moved at whim or are consistent, if he is incapable of understanding them?

No, I am not arguing against setting our children limits, for the simple reason that it would be impossible. What I am saying is we shouldn't set artificial and artful ones. If our child asks us for something which isn't harmful to him, which doesn't destroy the environment, which we can afford, which we have time to give him, let us not say "no" simply "in order to set him limits" or "to accustom him to being obedient".

If we have refused him something, and we see that his response is "disproportionate", could it be that we have misjudged the situation, could what we have refused him be much more important to him than we thought? Then let us reconsider our decision in the light of this new discovery: will he catch a horrible disease if he has his bath tomorrow instead of today? Will the world come to an end if we wait until his favourite cartoon is over before going for a walk? Will he freeze to death if he doesn't wear a coat?

If in the end we decide not to give in; if he has to go to school, finish his homework, turn the TV off this instant, will we be able to exercise our authority without being overbearing, to give orders without resorting to shouts or threats, to tolerate our child's frustration and accept that he obeys us grudgingly, not with a big smile on his face, like the good little boys and girls in the movies? It is well known that Napoleon's grenadiers "grumbled and followed him faithfully";[70] even he couldn't force them to obey without complaining.

Connected to the theme of limits is the widespread belief that small children practice a strange and exclusive activity known as "stretching the limits", exclusive because apparently no adult indulges in this.

For example, imagine a friend of yours drops by one afternoon. "Oh, what a lovely vase!" She picks it up, she admires it, it slips from her hands, and the antique porcelain vase (an heirloom from your grandmother) is smashed to smithereens. Why did your friend do that? Was she stretching the limits? If you don't punish her immediately, from now on she will smash any vase she can lay her hands on, and she will probably draw all over the walls and open all the gas knobs, because she will have lost all respect for you.

What nonsense! She dropped it by accident, she is very upset, she won't stop apologising even though you assure her she needn't worry, and she won't go near another vase for years.

But what if your daughter breaks the vase? What makes you think her reasons are any different?

The difference, in any case, is knowledge and experience. A two-year-old girl still doesn't know that porcelain is fragile and that plastic isn't; on top of which, she is incapable of staying still and clumsier with her hands. Of course, you have to teach her gradually which things she can play with and which not, and how to handle fragile objects with care. But at no time does your daughter think: "Let's see how far I can go. I'll break a vase, and see if I get away with it." You are the one who has been foolish enough to leave a priceless vase within reach of a two year-old girl. When you have children, valuable objects are placed out of reach or under lock and key, and they aren't taken out again until the youngest has been civilised. This is the perfect occasion to leave lying around all the awful presents people have given you, which you don't know how to get rid of.

What do you do if your daughter has just broken a priceless vase? Choose one of the following options:

a. Smack her hand.
b. Say: "Look what you've done now! I've told you 100 times to be careful! I'm sick and tired of you!"
c. Punish her by not taking her to the park.
d. Say: "I was very fond of that vase, it was very valuable and it was the only memento I had of my grandmother. I'm very upset now and it's all your fault, I hope you're pleased with yourself."
e. Say: "You'll have to pay for at least half of the vase, so you'll only get half your pocket money from now until Christmas."
f. Say: "Oh, what a shame, the vase is broken! You have to be terribly careful with them, they aren't toys. Come on, we'd better sweep up the pieces."
g. Say: "Don't worry; it's only an old vase."

Note that if your friend, neighbour, or sister-in-law had broken the vase, you wouldn't hesitate to choose 'g'. You would say it over and over again, while she apologised until she was blue in the face. Well, I think it is also the best choice for an eight-year-old girl. She is old enough to know that the vase is important, that she has to handle it with care, that you are hiding the fact that you are upset out of consideration. She is sad, ashamed and would do anything not to have broken the vase. There is no need for reproaches or lectures.

'E' is a popular choice for parents of older children, although I find it rather petty. You would never ask your friend for money, nor would you accept if she offered, even if she was earning a good salary. How can you ask your daughter for money when she is a minor and doesn't earn enough even to buy herself an ice-cream?

If it is your two-year-old daughter who breaks the vase, 'g' may be a bad choice. She might believe you and think there is no difference between breaking a porcelain vase and bursting a balloon. At that age, an answer like 'f' seems respectful, understandable and informative. Even so, keep your other ornaments in a safe place, because small children don't always understand things the first time round.

Permissiveness: the fear of freedom

> *I don't consider myself permissive at all.*
> Dr Spock

Benjamin Spock is the author of *Baby and Child Care*,[71] the most influential and best-selling book on parenting, which has sold tens of millions of copies since it was published in 1945. Dr Spock was also politically engaged, and demonstrated against America's involvement in the Vietnam War and in favour of nuclear disarmament. He has often been accused of being permissive, to the extent that in the prologue of the 1985 edition of his book, he felt obliged to defend himself:

> The accusation came for the first time in 1968, twenty-two years after the book came out, from a prominent clergyman who objected strongly to my opposition to the war in Vietnam. He said that my advice to parents to give "instant gratification" to their babies and children was what made these babies grow up to be irresponsible, undisciplined, unpatriotic adults . . . There is no instant gratification in this book.

This is true, the book doesn't speak of instant gratification. But first let us look at some of his other warnings:

> By about three or four months, it's a good idea for babies to get used to falling asleep in their own beds, without company. . . This is one way to prevent later sleep problems. . . If your child

starts out sleeping in your room, two to three months is a good age to move her out.

Furthermore, if the baby is ill or so anxious that he wants to spend the whole night in his parent's bed, Spock recommends that, besides consulting a doctor (such a desire must be pathological, of course), the parents go to the child's room in order to calm him down: "Sit by his cot in a relaxed way until he goes to sleep."

Parents may also allow their children into their bed in the mornings, for a cuddle, "so long as it doesn't make either parent uneasy, by stirring up sexual feelings". Feelings, which he attributes to "sexual advances" on the part of the child. Doesn't this strike you as incredibly twisted? The first thing that enters his head when a small child gets into his parents' bed in order to give them a kiss or jump up and down on the mattress, is that his parents may experience disturbing sexual feelings initiated moreover by their child. And yet, in many other situations in daily life, which are on the face of it more compromising, nobody notices such things. You won't find in any book warnings such as: "You may go to the beach providing that seeing half-naked bodies doesn't arouse in you sexual feelings", or "Of course taking public transport is more ecological than driving, but before you take the underground or the bus, ask yourself whether you aren't actually hoping to rub up against someone."

Dr Spock doesn't much favour picking children up or paying them much attention either, believing that it is unnecessary to pick the child up as soon as he awakes and that a child of a few months old can be spoiled by too much attention.

None of this differs much from what many other experts, old and new, have said. If I have devoted a section in this chapter, "Theories I do not share", to Dr Spock, it isn't because he is a bigger culprit than other authors – he isn't – but to demystify the false aura of permissiveness that surrounds him, which some parents may believe in. If making your child sleep on his own and hardly ever picking him up is permissive, what must one do to be "strict"?

Sooner protect than correct

> *Endeavour always to effect*
> *Honour and necessity in deed*
> *But sooner protect than correct*
> *Ere you not succeed*
> Guillen de Castro, YOUTHFUL DEEDS OF EL CID

Parents are usually advised never to back-pedal once they have taken a decision. If you give in once, you will always have to give in. Your child will no longer respect you. Under no circumstances must you listen to her protests or condescend to justify your authority to a child.

A father who gives in to a child's tantrum is, according to advocates of this myth, a bad father, a weak, pathetic creature who is doing harm to himself, and even more harm to his child, by showing her that through screaming and remonstrating she can get her own way. A father who gives in to a child's tantrum is (how should I describe it?) like an employer giving in to strikers or a government negotiating with demonstrators.

Oh, no, of course not. Employers must heed workers' rightful demands, and governments must listen to the people's voice as expressed in the sacred right to demonstrate. A government that never gave in, never backed down over its decisions, never negotiated and refused to listen to demonstrators, would be a dictatorial, anti-democratic, inefficient government. The world over, governments that are most able to negotiate, listen and give in enjoy the most steadfast loyalty and respect from their citizens, while the harshest governments, those that appear to be in control, are the ones that are always more at risk of being overthrown.

Why should it be any different with children? Why is what would be considered tyranny and bossiness in any other authority figure considered a virtue in parents?

Nicolaÿ[72] writes expertly about the dangers of giving in to a child:

> "Mum, can I have an apricot."
> "What are you saying, child. Are you crazy! You've just been ill, and the doctor said strictly no fruit, so get that idea out of your head!"
> The little girl protests.
> "It's no use protesting! I said no, do you hear?"
> The protests grow louder, and the tone changes: the mother is beginning to soften.
> "But, darling, you don't want to go on being ill, do you? Believe me, there's nothing more harmful than eating fruit in summer!"

The scene continues, with emotional blackmail and shouting on both sides, the mother offers her half an apricot, the child wants all of it, finally the mother gives her the whole apricot:

> "Here, have the bloody apricot; go on, how many more do you want, two, three? You can eat the whole lot if you want, see if I care, I hope you burst, it'll serve you right!"

Does the modern reader notice anything strange? For me several things stand out: what illness is this where eating apricots is forbidden? What is wrong with eating fruit in summer? Did they eat no fruit all summer?

Nicolaÿ was attempting to demonstrate the "terrible" effects of lack of discipline: the mother incapable of imposing her authority, the little girl "getting her own way". Nowadays, most would agree with the basic idea, but the example would probably be inverted: "Come on, eat your fruit, you know the doctor said it's very healthy and full of vitamins." "I don't want it!" "All right, don't eat fruit if you don't want to! And it'll serve you right if your teeth fall out or you go blind!"

Since the two mothers completely contradict one another,

at least one of them has to be wrong. They may even both be wrong. In the name of what moral or pedagogic principle should parents impose their opinion (even when it is misguided) and should the child obey (even when he is right)? Blind obedience to authority may appear logical to nineteenth-century subjects, but citizens of the twenty-first century should aspire to something more.

The mother in the story makes a few mistakes, but giving in isn't one of them. Her first mistake (for which she is not to blame, incidentally, as it is the doctor who advised her), is to imagine that a child can become ill from eating fruit. (Modern mothers commonly make the opposite mistake, also propagated by doctors, that children can become ill if they don't eat fruit.) Her second mistake is not giving in sooner. She was acting, it will be said, under intense pressure from the doctor, who had warned her of the serious dangers posed by apricots. But, in that case, she should never have given in. If you are absolutely convinced that something is seriously harmful for your child, you can't give in even if she throws 100 tantrums. Or would you allow your child to swallow bleach or throw herself from the balcony to stop her from crying? That mother didn't give in because she hoped her daughter would "burst", as she said out of annoyance, but precisely because she knew it wouldn't make her burst. Deep down, she knew the doctor's warning about the serious dangers of eating fruit in the summer was an exaggeration and that the danger (if any) was very slight. So why all the fuss if this wasn't a matter of life or death, if in the end it was so trivial? If you think you can give in, do so quickly and avoid arguments.

Her third mistake is not giving in gracefully. Instead of savage remarks like: "I hope you burst!", or more subtle, and perhaps more insidious, manipulations such as: "Here, have the apricot. But you know I'm very annoyed and above all disappointed. You've been a very naughty girl", what harm is there in being a little nicer, getting out of a fix and at the same time saving face and preserving your dignity? ("All right, have the apricot. I didn't know you liked them so much...")

Fernand Nicolaÿ was a French magistrate and thinker, author of a book called *Spoiled Children*,[72] which was a great success: the copy I came across is the twelfth Spanish edition, translated from the twentieth French edition. There is no publication date inside, and although the cover could be from the 1940s, the text gives the impression of being older, for there is no mention in it of cars, radios, televisions or aeroplanes... I found more information on the Internet. The French National Library catalogue contains fifteen of Nicolaÿ's works, published between 1875 and 1922, including three editions of *Spoiled Children* from 1890, 1891 and 1907. Only in the 1891 edition is there a reference to it being the eleventh edition.

Nicolaÿ insists his ideas aren't simple opinions, they are experimental science, for he has written down on a piece of paper a list of well-behaved children he knows, and another list of spoiled ones, "this list being lengthy, interminable", and has subsequently examined the methods of the different parents. He describes in great detail, and over several chapters, the trajectory of these ill-mannered children, whom he claims make up the majority of French men and women of his time.

At three years old, they show an "unshakable disobedience", "it is the child that dictates", he only eats what he pleases... At ten years old, "he is more insolent", "he shouts more loudly", and his parents daren't refuse him anything, he thinks he is special... At fifteen, "his primitive innocence has given way to an idiotic presumptuousness", he pokes fun at his parents' ignorance, he is rude... At twenty, "the house is run according to the master's whim", he is a useless wretch and a sponger. As an adult (over the age of twenty), he is "an incompetent wastrel, idle and ambitious, a callous libertine".

I have summarised in one paragraph over eighty pages, but the book is the same all the way through. The description of the spoiled three-year-old child is remarkably similar to that of many modern-day authors:

For the last few years, people have begun to notice in children a tendency to do whatever they want […]. We often hear people say: "Children have no 'respect' for anything these days". (Langis, 1996.)[2]

And here we have the crux of the matter, which is why I went to so much trouble in order to discover the date of Nicolaÿ's book. For the last few years? Surely not? The children Nicolaÿ is referring to, dear reader, aren't your children, they are your great-grandparents. Yes, your great-grandparents, whose great-great-grandparents spoiled them so horribly. Your great-grandfather then spoiled your grandfather who spoiled your father, and your father, became "an incompetent wastrel, idle and ambitious, a callous libertine", who in turn spoiled you. How do we account for all these myths ("We had more respect for our parents", "In the old days there was more discipline", "We couldn't get away with anything")? Yet, according to Nicolaÿ, the vast majority of children were already spoiled over 100 years ago.

No, we don't lose our children's respect by giving in to them, by negotiating, by acknowledging our mistakes; on the contrary we win it.

When we give in, we are teaching them how to give in.[44]

A long time ago, when I was thirteen or fourteen, my father scolded me for no reason. At any rate I have long forgotten the reason whatever it was. What I do remember very clearly was my deep resentment at such immense unfairness. I went to bed hurt and in tears, and then, to my amazement, my father came to say goodnight, and he apologised. A father apologising to his son! Isn't that the surest way to lose all authority over your son as well as his respect? On the contrary. At that moment all his sins, past present and future, were absolved.

A timely smack

> *Children are never too tender to be whipped: —*
> *like tough beefsteaks, the more you beat them*
> *the more tender they become.*
> Edgar Allan Poe, FIFTY SUGGESTIONS

> *I'm not particularly advocating spanking, but I think*
> *it is less poisonous than lengthy disapproval,*
> *because it cleans the air, for parent and child.*
> Dr Spock, BABY AND CHILD CARE

Many psychologists and educators have sung the praises of smacking.

In Spain, the number of young children physically abused by their parents rose from 2,600 in the year 2001 to 6,400 in the year 2005 (this is probably because more cases are reported and not due to an increasing problem). In that same period, between eight and sixteen children died at the hands of their parents. This data comes from the National Police Force and the Civil Guard, and was collected by the Queen Sofia Centre as part of a study on violence.[92] However, these data only include abuses serious enough to have been brought to police attention, and excludes cases dealt with by the regional police forces in the Basque Country and in Catalonia. In the United States 1,185 deaths were registered in 1995, which represented a 34 percent increase in a little over ten years.[73] And yet, a few random murders committed by teenagers unleash a wave of hysteria ("Are we raising monsters?"), as if it were children who habitually abused their parents. I heard one learned expert in a radio debate claim this was the result of State interference in the family arena, because a year earlier a law had been passed that banned hitting children. A timely smack would have prevented those crimes! An eight-year-old child whose parents give him a good smack learns that conflicts are resolved by violence, and that the strong can impose their views on the weak. I fail to see how these early lessons, and this shining example help prevent a child from becoming a teenage killer.

Let us examine a specific case. Jaime considers he is a good husband and a tolerant father, but some things make him lose his temper. Sonia is very difficult, she never does what she is told and she answers back. She "forgets" to make the bed, even when you remind her a dozen times. She is fussy about her food; if she doesn't like the look of something, she won't even try it. If you turn the TV off, she turns it back on without even looking at you. She takes money out of your purse without even bothering to ask. She constantly interrupts. When she gets angry (which happens a lot), she bursts into tears, runs to her room and slams the door. Sometimes she locks herself in the bathroom; at times like this, no amount of reasoning will calm her down. In fact, once, Jaime had to kick the door in to get her to come out. But what really infuriates Jaime is when she is disrespectful. Last night, for example, Sonia took paper from the desk to draw on. "I told you not to take paper from the desk without asking", Jaime told her. "Who do you think you are? I'll take as much paper as I want!", Sonia replied. Jaime gave her a smack, and shouted: "Don't speak to me like that. Apologise this instant!", but Sonia, far from admitting her mistake, stood up to him and replied insolently: "You're the one who should apologise!" Jaime gave her another smack, at which she screamed: "Asshole!", and ran off. Jaime had to make a supreme effort to stop himself from chasing after her. When this sort of thing happens, it is best to calm down and count to ten. Of course, Sonia will be confined to the house for the rest of the week.

That is the story. Now let us suppose that Sonia is seven years old and that Jaime is her father. How does it look to you? Isn't this one of those occasions when any reasonable person might "lash out"? Didn't that smack "clean the air", as Dr Spock so eloquently put it? What can those fanatics who banned smacking children do in a case like this? Will they drag the father before the courts for hitting his little girl who, incidentally, was asking for it? Isn't it preferable to let these problems be resolved in the family, without any outside interference? Perhaps you are thinking that with a few timely smacks this little girl would never have become so disobedient and mouthy. The situation seems typical of children spoiled by permissive parents, who don't know how to set clear limits, and who don't impose the necessary discipline: what is tolerated today elicits an exaggerated response tomorrow, and as a result the little girl is confused and unhappy.

And what if I told you, dear reader, that Sonia is in fact seventeen and that Jaime is her father? Does that change anything? Reconsider the story in the light of this new fact. Do you think she is perhaps too old for her father to be smacking her, turning the TV off or making her ask before taking a simple sheet of paper? Do you think it is appropriate for a father to kick down the bathroom door because his daughter has locked herself in there? Are you beginning to wonder whether this father is obsessive, tyrannical and violent, and that his daughter's response is reasonable and understandable?

And if so, why this difference? Let us reflect for a moment about the criteria you have used to judge this father and this daughter. Are young children required more than teenagers to respect adults' things, to remember and obey their parents' orders, uncomplainingly, with a smile on their face, to be nice and polite, however angry they are inside, to stay calm and not to cry or make a scene? Is shouting or hitting more harmful to teenagers than it is to young children? The law doesn't follow those criteria in the case of juveniles. On the contrary, the younger the child, the less responsible the judges deem him to be, and the lighter the sentence (if any). Who is right: the "interfering" State, which doesn't consider the child responsible for his actions, or the "reasonable and judicious" father, who corrects his child while the child is still young. Perhaps instead of social workers, educators, juvenile courts and reformatories, we should open high security prisons and bring back the use of torture for juvenile delinquents.

But there is still another, even more disturbing, possibility. What if I were to tell you that Sonia is twenty-seven and that Jaime is her husband? (No, I haven't cheated. Re-read the story and you will see that at no point did I mention that Sonia was Jaime's daughter.) Do you think it is normal for a husband to turn the TV off while his wife is watching it because "she's watched enough", or to order her to make the bed, or to make her eat everything on her plate, or to prohibit her from taking paper or to smack her? Do you still think Jaime is a good husband, but that Sonia is difficult and makes him lose his temper? Isn't it any husband's right to correct and mould his wife's character, resorting if necessary to punishment ("tough love")? Did she not swear before God and man to respect and obey her husband? Should the State intervene in a strictly private matter?

Why when you read the story for the first time did you think Sonia was a child? Well, precisely because Jaime shouted at her and hit her. Unconsciously, you thought: "If he treats her like that, she must be his daughter." It doesn't occur to us that she could be an adult, in the same way, when we read the words "racist attack" in a headline, it wouldn't occur to us to think that the victims might be Swedish.

Violence seems more acceptable when the victim is a child, and the younger the better.

Let us look at another example. Pedro, who is six, asks for chewing gum at the grocer's. Maite pretends not to have heard him. Pedro insists. "Can I have some chewing gum, please?" "No." "I want chewing gum!" "I said no!" "I want chewing gum!" "Look, you're getting on my nerves. I've told you ten times, you're not getting any chewing gum", Maite exclaims, grabbing the boy by the arm and dragging him out of the grocer's shop.

Who hasn't seen or experienced a scene like that? It is easy to imagine a mother ending up by losing her patience...

But what if Maite isn't the boy's mother? What if the

mother, dear reader, is you? You have sent your son Pedro out to the grocer's, a coin in his little hand, to buy some chewing gum (he doesn't even have to cross the road), and Maite, who works there, has treated him in this way. Wouldn't you lodge a complaint? You would never go into that shop again!

Violence against a child seems more acceptable when the aggressor is the parent or teacher than when it is a stranger. In fact, we would never allow a stranger to go up to our child in the street and hit him.

And which is more acceptable to the child? Violence coming from a stranger can be painful and frightening. But from your own parent! As well as pain and fear you feel surprise, confusion, betrayal and guilt (yes, guilt; it may seem incredible but children are inclined to think that if they get hit they must have done something wrong. Even those hit by an alcoholic parent feel guilt). A stranger only hurts your body; your parents can hurt your soul.

Now imagine your ten-year-old son has been in a fight at school. A jostle, a shove, a few exchanged insults and a tussle on the ground... End result: a boy in tears, his clothes dirty, and a scraped knee. Would you go to the school to lodge a complaint or to speak to the parents of the aggressors or the aggressors themselves? Probably not, unless the attacks were continuous, or your son was badly hurt. After all, "boys will be boys". Furthermore, many fathers, and quite a few mothers would tell their son to stop being a cry-baby and stand up to the bullies...

Wait a minute, did I say your ten-year-old son? I meant to say your thirty-year-old husband. A colleague at work laid him out flat after a quarrel, while their fellow workers laughed and jeered: "Give him what for!" Is there any difference?

Of course there is. We find that kind of behaviour unacceptable. And it doesn't need to be repeated on a daily basis, or for any bones to be broken for it to be unacceptable. I have seen people suing for lesser offences. If an adult lodges a complaint for aggression, he isn't considered a sneak, he is defending his rights. Whereas children are subject to a law of silence, as ruthless as that of the mafia, and fellow pupils and even teachers will most likely despise anyone who complains.[74]

We can invent a thousand excuses to hide this reality, but the fact is our society condemns violence, except when the victim is a child. If the victim is a child, and the aggressor another child, a teacher, or especially a parent, we will tolerate and sometimes applaud incredible amounts of violence. David Finkelhor, an American sociologist, who has carried out in-depth studies of family violence and abuse, points out three main reasons why children are so often the objects of violence:[75]

1. Children are weak and dependant of adults.
2. The law doesn't do enough to protect them, and society doesn't condemn acts of aggression.
3. Children can't choose with whom they associate: they can't change parents, school or neighbourhood whenever they want.

Am I saying then that we can never, under any circumstances, hit a child? Yes, that is precisely what I am saying. In that case how are we to enforce discipline? Imagine your child does exactly the same thing in fifteen years' time. You won't be able to hit him because he will be stronger than you (that, let us be honest, is the main reason why we don't hit older boys). So how will you deal with the situation? You had better start practising.

I agree with Spock[71] when he says that some parents resort to even more harmful forms of violence, such as humiliation, constant shouting, ridicule or derision. As in all things, there are degrees, and daily insults and ridicule can be worse than the odd gentle smack. But that argument doesn't wash with me as a justification for smacking.

Should the police arrest parents who hit their children? Or, in a broader sense, are we bad parents because we have occasionally hit our children, or because we have often hit them? Will my child be traumatised because once, twelve years ago, I lost my temper and hit him?

Of course the police and the law must intervene in cases of serious violence and cruelty; and other slightly less serious cases will fall within the area of psychiatry and social services. But it is equally true that it would be difficult to find a parent who hasn't at one time or another raised a hand to or shouted at their child.

Couples, relatives, friends and colleagues, also occasionally (or repeatedly) quarrel bitterly, insult or ridicule each other, and even come to blows, and yet they manage to make up and carry on as before. Undoubtedly, in many cases of minor aggression, both within and outside the family, the intervention of the police or the law would only aggravate things, and make it more difficult to come to an amicable agreement.

In my opinion, it is the justification of violence against children that distinguishes it from other types of violence in our society, and is an unspeakable disgrace. A large section of public opinion, as well as countless experts and intellectuals, who in other respects are educated, kind and understanding, maintain that a "timely smack" is not only acceptable, but recommendable: a useful "educational" tool that helps the victim become a better person. The victim is told: "It's for your own good", or even, the height of shamelessness: "It hurts me more than it hurts you." No one, or no one living in a democracy at the beginning of the twenty-first century at any rate, would dare justify violence in this way if the victim were an adult.

We needn't look as far as those extreme cases reported in the press, of cigarette burns and broken bones. Every day children are hit for "answering back", they are shouted at, ridiculed and insulted for perfectly innocent deeds, punished because of accidents or involuntary mistakes, locked for hours in their rooms, which become punishment cells, forced to eat food they have puked up, or forbidden from going outside to run around in the fresh air or play. And all in accordance with unwritten laws and rules, norms that are often invented after the fact, and meted out by a single person who acts as law enforcer, witness, judge and executioner, with no written document, no defence, no possibility of appeal (protest generally leads to a stiffer sentence). If all of this were to happen not in a home, but in a prison, and if the victims weren't children but criminals and terrorists, there would be appeals before parliament.

I suggest that we put an end to this justification – that we stop thinking the way we act and begin acting the way we think.

If at any time "we lash out" at our child, let us do exactly what we would do if we had lashed out at a colleague or an adult member of our family:

- Try our best never to let it happen again.
- Acknowledge that we have done something wrong and feel ashamed.
- Apologise to the victim.

An expert on hitting children

I couldn't end this chapter without examining the arguments of some advocates of smacking. There are the traditional ones Miller[35] quotes from:

> The blows you administer should not be merely playful ones but should convince him that you are his master. [...] But you must pay especial heed that in chastising him you not allow yourself to be overcome by anger. For the child will be sharp-witted enough to perceive your weakness and regard as a result of anger what he should deem a meting out of justice (J.G. Krüger, 1752.)

Among contemporary authors, I have found none as convincing as Dr Christopher Green, a Northern Irishman living in Australia who wrote a book with the revealing title: *Toddler Taming*.[76]

Green begins by saying that "in no way can I condone beating, excessive punishment, violence or child abuse". He goes on to accuse "some anti-corporal punishment lobbyists" of

> [...] using their position and misinformation to cause unnecessary concern in the majority of good parents who are not averse to the occasional smack.

It isn't clear whether these "good parents" are good in spite of or because of smacking. It is remarkable the way guilt has been reversed here: the victim isn't the child whose own father has smacked him, it is the poor father who has been "unnecessarily concerned" by misinformed lobbyists. Might not a "timely" dose of "unnecessary concern" be good for parents' education?

Green goes on to explain a few cases in which smacking is wrongly used: lack of consistency (the parent feels remorseful about hitting his son and gives in); the straw that breaks the camel's back (the parent puts up with "a long series of annoyances" and then blows up over something trivial); the danger that the child may hit his parent back; the child that remains indifferent:

> Some toddlers have the most amazing theatrical talent. When smacked they stand stoically like Rambo under interrogation, look you in the eye and with the dumbest of dumb insolence, say: "That didn't hurt!" Of course it hurt but they know this reaction will infuriate and punish the smacker for laying a finger on one so important.

We are speaking of children under four years old. Children at that age (and also older), who receive an occasional smack, respond with shock and disbelief, frustration and uncontrollable sobbing. A child who holds back his tears and says: "That didn't hurt", must have been "toughened" by dozens of smacks. Once again the victim is at fault: the child who has been hit is "insolent", a consummate actor, thinks he is very important and "punishes".

Are we to understand that a father who repeatedly hits his three-year-old child isn't insolent, a consummate actor or bigheaded, but on the contrary, kind, sincere and humble?

If you don't cry when hit, you are insolent: but watch out, because if you do cry you are manipulative, as Dr Green warns in another passage:

> "Every time I raise my voice to discipline, he disintegrates into floods of tears." This is a common situation where correct and appropriate discipline backfires leaving the parents punished, confused and feeling guilty [...] They know they have a losing hand, but use tears to trump their parents.

The use of the word "trump", with its dual meaning of playing a trump card and deceiving, exemplifies Dr Green's generous opinions about children. Thus, dear reader, if your father hits you, don't cry too hard or you will make him feel guilty, and don't refrain from crying as this will have the same lethal effect. Nice children, who are always careful not to cause their parents any psychological trauma, respond to smacks with a quick, quiet cry, which expresses a deep understanding of their parent's concern and a resolution to change their ways.

Dr Green goes on to explain the correct way to smack children. (Yes, dear reader, here and in other civilised countries, we publish manuals on how to hit children, and such books haven't been taken off the market, or their authors denounced. Can you imagine the uproar it would cause if the police brought out a handbook called *Taming Suspects*, explaining the correct way to hit a prisoner?) Green claims it is best to smack young children, two-year-olds, and that a smack has an immediate effect, it establishes clear limits, prevents an escalation of the conflict, ends an impasse, and is a very useful way of discouraging children from doing dangerous things.

For example: a child begins climbing the balcony balustrade.

What better way to prevent him from doing this again, says Green, than a "hard smack"? Well, I can think of several. In the first place, a child of two or three is incapable of climbing up a balcony balustrade without a serious lapse in security having occurred: there shouldn't be any flower pots that can be scaled, balconies with horizontal railings should be outlawed, and a child that young should never be left alone on a balcony. If we are distracted for a second, the next thing we might see is our child climbing the balustrade. When we hit him we aren't "teaching" him, we are punishing him for something for which we know we are to blame. However, since we are only human, and therefore flawed, sooner or later our child will put himself in danger when we aren't looking: whether on a balcony, crossing a street, in the kitchen or by sticking his fingers in a socket. Obviously it wouldn't be enough in a case like that simply to say: "Darling, you really mustn't touch the gas knobs!" But the logical, natural response of any parent, which is to look very serious, yell at him to stop, tell him the kitchen is "ouch" and quickly remove him from it closing the door behind you, is enough to make any child who isn't accustomed to being smacked burst into tears. If the child is grown up enough (aged four, say), this will be enough to stop him from touching the gas knobs ever again. If the child is one and a half, you had best be vigilant, because, smack or no smack, he is probably too young to understand that gas knobs can be dangerous.

Another expert on smacking, a Spaniard this time, is Dr Castells, a child psychiatrist.[77] He suggests, among other things, a truly original use for smacking:

> When your child starts crying inconsolably for no reason, it is preferable to provide him with one, for instance by giving him a good smack.

Do children cry for no reason? Have you, dear reader, ever cried for no reason? The child cries because he is cold, hungry, in pain, tired, frustrated or angry, but in any event he cries about something. The closest a human being gets to "crying for no reason" occurs in depressive illnesses; and as far as I know, the usual treatment for depression in adults isn't smacking. Just in case, if I ever feel depressed, I will be very careful not to visit the clinic of a certain psychiatrist…

Parents are being told to ignore and condemn their child's tears, not to try to calm him, console him, cuddle him, listen to him, see whether anything is the matter, or at least to offer him some contact and company. Why worry about your child's suffering, why try to share it with him, when it is much easier to give him a smack and everyone will be happy.

> If your son does not want to learn because it is your will, if he cries with the intent of defying you, if he does harm in order to offend you, in short, if he insists on having his own way: Then whip him well till he cries so: Oh no, Papa, oh no! [Kruger, quoted by Miller.][35]

Those who prefer the more difficult path: using words instead of violence, will enjoy another, very different book by Cubells and Ricart (a paediatrician and child psychologist respectively).[44] They start from a basic premise:

> We must also forget the cliché that the child cries because he wants to. In order to cry it is necessary to feel something.

Surprisingly, advocates of smacking often feel the need to clear their reputation:

> First let me state unequivocally that I am not a smacking enthusiast. (Green.)[76]

> Having said this, the reader must not think we are sadists and out-and-out child-beaters. (Castells.)[77]

God forbid! We wouldn't have thought it for a moment... One of the most terrible aspects of violence against children is the ease with which it is reproduced in generation after generation. Castells describes this clearly (for it is a fact well-known to scientists, and as a psychiatrist he can't be ignorant of it):

> Similarly, we are aware that some parents are fervent advocates of corporal punishment because they themselves were persistently beaten as children.[77]

Yes, children who have been mistreated frequently become abusive parents. There are several factors which contribute to perpetuating this vicious circle. On the one hand, the child grows up unaware of any other way of doing things, any other way of bringing up children. He also grows up with psychological problems resulting from the abuse to which he has been subjected, problems such as aggressiveness or the inability to empathise with others' suffering. But, also, and perhaps most importantly, the child grows up needing to defend his parents. Children love their parents to distraction, and feel obliged to defend them.[35] Everything my parents did was good. If I don't hit my children, it is as if I were telling my parents they were wrong to hit me. On the next page, Castells, with absolute filial devotion, incurs the exact same error he has just attributed to others:

> All – or the vast majority – of us have received the odd resounding slap from our parents, which, intriguingly, we recall with affection and a sense of nostalgia now they are no longer here to dispense them.[77]

Theophile Gautier expressed this sentiment long before in his beautiful description of the young Baron Sigognac's sorrow (*Captain Fracasse*):

His father's attention, which in spite of everything he missed, had amounted to little more than a few kicks up the backside or a command for him to be flogged. At such moments, he felt a terrible longing, and would gladly have received one of his father's admonishments, the memory of which brought tears to his eyes, for a kick from father to son is still a relationship . . .

A relationship, indeed. Children are so desperate for contact and attention from their parents they will even accept abuse as proof of love for want of anything better. Some children, who are unable to get enough "healthy" attention in the normal way, will seek attention in abnormal, pathological, ways. They are "bad", rebellious children, who are apparently "asking for it". Some parents explain the smack by saying: "He was begging for it." Do you think your child would ask for a smack if he were able or knew how to ask for something else, if he felt capable of receiving something else, if he were able (in the most serious cases) to conceive of the existence of something else?

I, too, hope my children will miss me one day with tears in their eyes, or that they will remember me with affection. But I hope not because of a kick or a smack. What indelible memory would you like to leave your child?

Rewards and punishments

> So Eppie was reared without punishment.
> George Eliot, SILAS MARNER

Many who are against slapping still defend other forms of punishment: the docking of privileges (no pudding, no TV), punishment as a natural consequence ("If you don't treat your toys properly, I'll take them away")... American society appears particularly obsessed with punishment, or at least in their sitcoms one is surprised to see teenage boys, almost grown men, say quite naturally: "I've been bad, I know: I'll be grounded for two weeks."

I don't think children need punishment in order to learn, in the same way we adults don't need it. Children want to make their parents happy, and they try their hardest (although sometimes they don't know how). The child who knows he has done wrong will try to avoid doing it again without any need for punishment. And the child who doesn't know only needs telling. If he disagrees, if he genuinely believes he is in the right, punishing him won't change his mind. On the contrary, he will feel angry and humiliated, and will do the same thing again at the first opportunity. The most punishment can teach you is how to do certain things in an underhand way so as not to be caught. That isn't moral conscience, it is pure hypocrisy.

It is perfectly possible to educate a child without punishment and without the threat of punishment.

I don't much like rewards either. Naturally, this is another level entirely. Of course any child prefers a thousand rewards to a single punishment.

The fact is a mother asked me once: "How can I offer my son a reward without it seeming like blackmail?" This made me reflect. A reward does indeed appear suspiciously like blackmail. "If you get good grades, I'll buy you the video console" is no different to: "If you get bad grades, you won't get the video console."

Actually, for a child there is no greater reward than his parent's approval (and no punishment worse than their disapproval), and in that sense reward is natural and inevitable. We can't help congratulating him on getting good grades, or admiring his lovely drawings or thanking him for helping lay the table. And if he tears the pages out of the encyclopaedia or hits a smaller child, we can't help showing our disapproval; even if we try not to shout at him, our child will know he has done something wrong, something he shouldn't have done.

I am not suggesting we use approval as a "weapon" with which to manipulate our children. When I tell my daughter she has written a good story, I am not thinking: "My approval will act as a positive reinforcer of desirable behaviour", or "It will stimulate her creative tendencies." I am simply thinking: "What a good story my daughter has written."

We should also be careful to separate approval and affection. We may be more or less pleased with what they do, but this shouldn't make us love them any more or less. Obviously, we must never say (or think): "I don't love you because you've been naughty" (sadly, we often say this even though we don't think it). But it is equally dangerous to say: "I love you because you've been very good", because it probably isn't true. If you love your children unconditionally, if you will love your children no matter what they do, why hide it, why make them think your love is conditional?

But aside from approval, the conscious and deliberate use of rewards and promises to influence our children's behaviour has, in my opinion, two huge disadvantages:

- The nature of the reward. "If you get good grades, we'll go to the beach this summer." And if you don't, will we spend the whole summer languishing at home? "If you tidy your room, I'll give you a bag of sweets." But don't sweets rot your teeth? How can we give him a reward we know is bad for him? What will the reward be in fifteen years' time, cigarettes or alcohol? "If you help me with the dusting, I'll buy you a book." But isn't it good for him to read? How can we justify not buying him a book? And this goes for all other possible rewards. All the things you can and should give to him you will give out of love, unconditionally. And you don't want to become a frenetic consumer, offering him useless and unnecessary rewards.
- Corruption. The very value of a moral action is tainted and degraded when rewards come into play. I take my children to the park because I know they like scampering about, because I enjoy watching them, because I spend

all day at work and they all day at school and I want to be with them at the weekends… So, am I going to spoil everything by saying: "As you've been good, I'll take you to the park"? Why hide my love, why pretend I am acting selfishly, like an employer who offers incentives to workers in order to increase production? My daughter has been very sweet to her baby cousin, she looked after him and let him play with her toys. She did it out of affection, because she loves her cousin and likes to see him happy; she swells with pride at having done the right thing… But had I said to her yesterday, "If you look after your baby cousin, I'll buy you a video game", would she still be able to feel proud? Did she look after her cousin because she loves him or did she tolerate him because of the money? Now she doubts her own motives, because I first doubted her.

Reward isn't a step forward on the path to education, it is a step backwards in the face of true generosity, which is unselfish and unconditional.

This is why I like to use words carefully. "If you finish your homework, we'll go to the cinema" sounds conditional, like blackmail; I prefer to say: "We're going to the cinema this afternoon, so hurry up and finish your homework."

Looking for problems

> *Papa talks enough of my defects, and shows enough*
> *scorn of me, to make it natural I should doubt myself.*
> *I doubt whether I am not altogether as worthless as*
> *he calls me, frequently; and then I feel so cross and*
> *bitter, I hate everybody! I am worthless, and bad*
> *in temper, and bad in spirit.*
> Emily Brontë, WUTHERING HEIGHTS

The Eyberg Behavioural Child Inventory (ECBI) is a questionnaire designed to detect behavioural problems in children,[78] in which parents are asked to evaluate their children in thirty-six different areas, for example: "Has poor table manners", "Whines", "Refuses to obey until threatened with punishment"...

The father or mother must assess the frequency with which their child carries out such atrocities (Never, Seldom, Sometimes, Often, Always), and they must also state whether they consider this behaviour to be a problem in their child. When the parents identify thirteen or more problems, it is because the child is suffering from a "behavioural disorder". Thus it was determined, in a study in the north of Spain, that 17 percent of children between the ages of two and thirteen had behavioural problems, and that the use of this questionnaire in paediatric clinics was very helpful. In theory, "behavioural disorder" is a psychiatric illness that requires specialised attention, yet it is doubtful that there are enough professionals to look after such a large number of "mentally ill" children.

The astute reader will have already appreciated the many problems involved in this type of "diagnosis".

Firstly, the doctor doesn't observe the child's behaviour at first hand, nor is he speaking to a neutral observer, he is speaking with the child's parents. If there is any conflict, the parents are an interested party and can't be considered impartial. What the questionnaire is in fact assessing is not the child's behaviour, but his parent's opinion of that behaviour. It isn't the same thing saying: "Sir, your child has a serious behaviour disorder" and saying: "Sir, you have a very low opinion of your child."

Secondly, this method attributes all the problems to the child. It is the child who shouts too much, who is disobedient or who cries a lot. There must be some parents who shout at their children too much, make them cry all the time with their insults and smacks, overwhelm them with too many demands and orders that are impossible to obey. And yet this questionnaire discovered none. How strange!

For example, to the statement: "Refuses to obey until is threatened with punishment", the normal response of parents should be: "I don't know, we've never threatened our child." In the Criminal Code of some countries, uttering threats is a crime or misdemeanour. If a husband were to say: "My wife refuses to obey me until I threaten to punish her", we would all think he had a behavioural problem. But if a mother or father says the same thing about their child, we think it is the child who is "problematic".

Thirdly, many (I would say most) of the points in the questionnaire offer more than dubious evidence of behavioural disorders:

Dawdles in getting dressed.

Define "dawdles". A serious questionnaire would have specified, for example: "He takes more than twelve minutes to put on his underwear, shirt and trousers." As it is, the judgement depends on the arbitrary criteria of the parents. At all events, many adults are guilty of this "behavioural disorder".

Whines.

This is rare in thirteen-year-olds, but don't all two- or five-year-olds cry?

Refuses to eat food presented.

Many people leave food on their plates in restaurants and no one seems to care. There are three possible reasons why a child refuses to eat what is put in front of him: there is too much food on the plate (that is, he isn't hungry), he doesn't like the food (I won't eat what I don't like either, how about you?), or he is ill and has no appetite.

Constantly seeks attention.

Young children need constant attention and therefore it is normal and healthy for them to seek it.

Gets angry when doesn't get own way.

Really? So do I! Maybe I have a screw loose and I didn't know it. Don't you get angry when you don't get what you want? "I'm so happy! I failed my exam, my girlfriend left me, I lost at bowling and I got a parking ticket. I haven't had this much fun in ages." If getting angry when we don't get our own way is a sign of mental illness, maybe we should all go to the asylum.

Is overactive or restless.

Anyone who has children knows this is perfectly normal. If your child can keep still for more than five minutes, maybe you ought to take him to the doctor.

Argues with parents about rules.

Hold on, aren't we living in a democracy? Arguing about rules is a right; it's called "participation". In order to grow up to be good citizens, and to be able to argue about rules with those in government it is necessary for children to practise at home.

Interrupts.

Interrupting people when they are talking is rude, but it is crucial when taking part in a radio or television debate. How often do we parents interrupt our children, how often do we grow impatient with their mumbling, how often do we cut them short: "Stop babbling", "Can't you see we're talking?", "I said 'no' and I mean 'no'", "Pleading won't get you anywhere"…?

Children learn from our example.

Wets the bed.

Bedwetting isn't a behavioural disorder, it is a normal variation in the pattern of a child's development. It has long been shown to be unrelated to any type of psychological problem.

Verbally fights with brothers and sisters.

Sibling rivalry is completely normal, and often the best thing a parent can do is to stay out of it.[79]

Has poor table manners.

Does anyone seriously believe that putting your elbows on the table or making slurping noises when you eat your soup justifies seeing a psychologist?

Fails to finish tasks or projects.

What of it! Most Gothic cathedrals are unfinished.

The severity of parental judgement when considering whether their child has a "behavioural problem" is surprising and worrying. Accordingly, 6 percent of parents affirm that their child "refuses to do chores when asked" always or often, while 52 percent say this happens "sometimes"; and yet 29 percent consider this a problem. That is to say, a large number of parents think that refusing to do chores "sometimes" already constitutes a problem. Similarly, only 5 percent "tease or provoke other children" always or often, yet 13 percent of parents see this as a problem; only 5 percent "fail to finish tasks or projects" always or often, yet 16 percent of parents see this as a problem; only 6 percent "have temper tantrums" always or often, and yet 21 percent of parents see this as a problem. Only in two of the sections, "Is overactive or restless" and "Wets his bed", did the opposite occur: some parents say their child does these things always or often but they don't see it as a problem (showing they have sounder judgement than the author of the questionnaire).

Isn't it possible that the constant repetition of negative remarks about children ends up degrading our perception of our own children?

Throw enough dirt and some will stick

> *[...] given the wanton corruption of youth in our times [...]*
> Margarita de Valois (1492–1549), THE HEPTAMERON

Many adults resort to stereotypes, insults and systematic vilification when speaking of children. This is often done in a jocular, almost "affectionate" way (he's a "little monster", "a little bully", "a positive nuisance"), but the damage is already done: parents are given the idea that their children are against them, and don't deserve to be respected as people. Let us consider a few specific examples:

As soon as put to bed, the little rascal starts to whinge.[15]

The "little rascal" is ten months old, yet his behaviour is considered not only conscious and calculated but also morally reprehensible. The choice of words isn't accidental: the baby doesn't begin to wail ("to express pain or sorrow by prolonged piteous cries", according to the dictionary), much less to weep ("to moan, to sob and to shed tears as an expression of painful emotion"), but to whinge ("to whine, to complain peevishly"). Perhaps he has good reason to complain!

Let us consider some more insults:

Toddlers are negative, show little sense and totally lack appreciation of the rights of others.[76]

Do you think I am exaggerating? Try replacing "toddlers" for "blacks" or "women" and tell me what you think then.

Ten percent of the [children in] the study group were little terrorists.[76]

This is a very serious accusation. Replace "children" with "trade unionists", "Catalans", "customers", "civil servants" or any other term referring to adults and you could receive a complaint against you for slander.

Make their mothers feel inferior. Little children have an incredible
ability to demoralise their mothers. Many will act as complete angels when in the care of others, reserving their demonic side exclusively for their parents.[76]

What a surprise! The fact is we all behave better with people we don't know than with our own family, without any need for insults or exaggerations such as "demonic". You will put up with slights from your colleagues, not to mention your employers, which would lead to an argument with your spouse.

We complain less about the food in a restaurant than at home (and we would never complain about the food at a friend's house). Those readers who are fathers and old enough to have been called up for mandatory military service, where were you most likely to do a good job of making your bed, to sweep and wash the floors without argument, where did you obey promptly and with a smile: at home or in the army? Does that mean you respected your sergeant more than your mother? Of course not, you were simply more afraid of him. In Spain there have been many more strikes and demonstrations under the socialist government than under Franco. Does that mean workers were happier under Franco? The fact is we protest more when we have more hope of gaining something by it, not when we are most wretched. We protest more when we feel accepted and loved. As Bowlby puts it:[80]

Thanks to the emotional bond linking child to parent and parent to child, children always behave in a more babyish way with their parents than with other people. [...] This is true even in the bird world. Young finches quite capable of feeding themselves will at once start begging for food in an infantile way if they catch sight of their parents.

Even Freud wasn't short of disapproval:

Too much maternal affection may be harmful to the child, it may hasten his sexual development, create bad habits, and render him incapable, in later stages of his life, of renouncing love in the short term or of being satisfied with partial love. Children with an insatiable demand for their mother's affection present the clearest symptoms of future anxiety. On the other hand, neuropathic fathers are, broadly speaking, more inclined to give their children excessive affection, thus awakening in them, before anyone else and with their caresses, a tendency to subsequent neurotic illnesses.[81]

Insulting parents is only a step away from insulting children, and so if you are affectionate towards your children you are a neuropath.

"No", the reader will say, "Freud only refers to people as neuropaths when they show excessive affection, not when they show a normal amount of affection." Very well, but what constitutes excessive affection? For many in our society, holding a child in your arms is already too much affection.

Freud isn't the only one who ridicules parents who are

"excessively" affectionate towards their children:

> Taking him out of his cot when he should be sleeping isn't a sign
> of affection but rather of stupid ignorance.[33]

This is how Dr Green describes his method of letting children
cry in order to teach them to go to sleep:

> Leave them crying for 5 minutes if you are average, 10 minutes if
> you are tough, 2 minutes if you are delicate and 1 minute if you
> are fragile. The length of crying depends on the the tolerance of
> parents and how genuinely upset the child becomes.[76]

That is to say, parents who don't want to let their child cry
are delicate, fragile and even lacking tolerance (intolerant!);
because in an amazing distortion of language, "tolerance" here
means the ability to listen to your own child cry without turning
a hair. Even if we were to concede that letting your child cry is
morally acceptable (something I refuse to concede!), wouldn't it
be more logical to adapt the length of time the child cries to his
own stamina rather than to that of his parents? (Let an average
child cry for five minutes, a delicate one for two minutes, a fragile
one…) But of course, Dr Green isn't concerned with the possible
suffering of a tiny baby, only with that of a twenty- or thirty-year-
old adult.

Sphincter control

One of our human rights that isn't commonly written about,
but which is nevertheless widely respected, is the right to
defecate when we want. Sometimes, of course, we feel the
urge during a social event, or when there is no toilet nearby,
and we are obliged to hold it in (and we all know how hard
that is). We also know how hard it is to defecate when we don't

want to (the typical "Go to the loo before we leave, because you won't be able to afterwards"). Can you imagine the owner of a factory forcing all his employees to go to the toilet between eleven and eleven fifteen in order to save time? Doesn't it seem more grotesque than humiliating, wouldn't there be an outcry, wouldn't it appear in the press?

If the idea of forcing an adult to go to the toilet at eleven forty-five or prohibiting him from going at thirteen twenty-eight appears ludicrous to us, then trying to force a baby to do the same should appear even more ludicrous. Our nine- or eighteen-month-old daughter doesn't soil her pants in order to upset us, or because she is wicked, or because there is something wrong with her; she does it because she is normal, because it is normal for babies of that age not to be able to control their sphincters. And if we sit our five- or fifteen-month-old daughter on a potty and nothing happens, we don't think she is trying it on, or being naughty, or that we should take her to a psychiatrist; we simply think that she is normal, that she doesn't know how to use a toilet yet. In fact, at five months old it wouldn't surprise us if she fell into the potty.

And yet there was a time, believe it or not, when people forced (or tried to force) nine- and five-month-old babies to use a potty. In 1941 Dr Ramos, referring to babies in their second trimester (i.e. between three and six months), said:

> Controlling the natural acts of defecation and urination is also a powerful means of education. After three months the mother will place the child on the potty at the time when he usually defecates [...] and if he fails to do so, it is acceptable, for a few days only, to apply a cocoa butter or glycerine suppository with the aim of making him associate the idea of "potty" with "doing number two".[37]

Did you notice here that sphincter control isn't an end in itself, but rather a means to an end? The child isn't being taught to do a poo in the potty, on the contrary: defecation is being controlled in order to train the child. Preventing the child from soiling himself is only a secondary aim. The primary aim is to train the child, that is to say, to teach him to obey, to bend to his parent's will. Anyone who has been taught to obey as ridiculous a command as "do a poo this instant" will obey future commands without question or protest. Freud already explained this quite clearly in 1905:

> One of the surest premonitions of later eccentricity or nervousness is when an infant obstinately refuses to empty his bowel when placed on the chamber by the nurse and reserves this function at its own pleasure.[81]

That is to say, an infant (let us assume this refers to a child under twelve months) who doesn't do a poo when his parents tell him, but who does it when he feels like it, is "refusing" to obey, "saving" this dubious pleasure, challenging his parents' authority, and showing clear symptoms of future abnormality and neurosis. According to Freud, all children who continue using nappies after they are one year old will be (or already are) neurotic. With good reason we say: "there are more crazy people than usually suspected!"

Why were Freud, Ramos and many others so convinced they were right? Did any of them see a child of under a year old using a potty successfully? Did they know some neurotics who had had problems with toilet training, and therefore concluded there is a link between the two things?

Indeed, the method worked with many children. Some babies defecate every day at the same hour, and if you put them on the potty at that precise hour, bingo! Through repetition, the child has come to associate the potty with doing a poo, and in the end this has created a conditioned reflex. The classic example of the conditioned reflex is Pavlov's famous dog, which was made to listen to a bell each time he was given food. In the end, hearing the bell was enough to make him start salivating ("his mouth watered"). The conditioned reflex is unconscious and doesn't require any intelligence (which the dog doesn't have), or free will (the dog can't salivate at will, only when he hears the bell).

If the association between sitting on the potty and doing a poo didn't occur of itself, it was helped along with a glycerine suppository or a laxative, which usually triggers defecation within minutes. Also, it is well known that the cold causes small children to urinate, so that simply having their trousers pulled down is likely to make them go.

But there were, of course, many children who didn't acquire this conditioned reflex, who wouldn't do a poo when ordered. Nowadays, grandmother, the woman next door, the nurse, the paediatrician and books tell inexperienced parents: "What do you expect? They are too young at that age to control their sphincters" and the parents say: "Oh, all right!", and put the potty away until next year, and that is that. There is nothing wrong with those children, and obviously they won't turn into neurotics.

Yet eighty years ago, when a six-month old child didn't do a poo in the potty, neighbours grandmothers, paediatricians, books and psychiatrists told parents: "I don't believe it, he is trying it on", "Maybe he is ill", "The same thing happened to a cousin of mine and he ended up in a lunatic asylum", "You have to keep trying", "This child needs taking in hand . . ." The beleaguered parents didn't give up, they would sit the child on the potty for hours ("You're not moving from there until you've done a poo."). They shouted, threatened, punished, ridiculed the child ("A big boy like you still in nappies!"), took him to the doctor, gave him laxatives, douches, and punished him by plunging his bottom into boiling water (there are still books describing the scalding this produced)... No wonder some of those poor children ended up neurotic. The prediction was fulfilled, and neighbours and paediatricians exclaimed: "I told you the child would come to a bad end if you didn't potty-train him before he was one", and Freud (like almost everyone in his time) confused cause and effect. They had no notion that it was their very attempts to "train" the child that had produced his neuroses. Fortunately, more and more doctors began to realise what the real problem was, and in the 1970s Dr Blancafort expressed perfectly the scientific thinking then (and now):

> Before twelve months it is useless and sometimes counterproductive to try to "train" a child to control his physiological needs properly. […] Children need to be educated, not "trained" as if they were animals. Indeed, that is the only thing stubborn, obsessive mothers would achieve: training their child, but at the cost of forcing him to spend hours on a potty. This would become a genuine ordeal for the little fellow, often producing an attitude of refusal and rejection, when not of outright terror. […] It is usual for children to be able to exercise complete control over these needs around the age of two.[82]

I agree completely. I have only one criticism of Dr Blancafort: instead of acknowledging that doctors and psychiatrists got this wrong, he blames "stubborn, obsessive mothers". Poor mothers. They were simply following advice given to them by paediatricians and psychiatrists thirty years earlier.

Aren't we lucky that raising children is now a science, and cruel practices such as potty training three month olds no longer exist? Except that they do, as similar cruel practices are used for "training" children to go to sleep. One day, when we realise that letting children cry at night and forcing them to sleep without their mothers for the first few years of their lives "is useless and sometimes counterproductive", and that such methods "train" but do not "educate", we will blame "stubborn obsessive mothers". As if it were their idea.

When and how to stop using nappies

People say "learning sphincter control", and this makes parents slightly uneasy. Because learning implies teaching. How do you teach a child sphincter control, whatever that is? And who is supposed to do the teaching?

No one. Learning not to wet oneself, like learning to walk, to sit down, to talk, are things that require no studying or teaching. There are ten-year-old children, and adults, who can't read or play the piano because no one has ever taught them. For them to learn, their parents have to do something (teach their child themselves or find a teacher or a school). But there is no such thing as a ten-year-old who doesn't know how to walk, sit down or talk, or who will wet herself (when awake). All healthy children (and a large number of unwell ones) are able to control when they pee (during the day) and do a poo by the age of four, or well before.

And so, the question isn't: "How should I go about teaching my daughter to use the toilet?", because your daughter will learn whether you teach her "well" or "badly" or not at all. The question is: "How can I prevent my daughter from suffering while she learns to use the toilet?" And the answer is: "The best way is by doing nothing." Or as little as possible.

When parents do something, when they sit their child on the potty at a specific time, when they make her sit there until she has produced something, when they tell her off if she soils herself, the child will in the long run also learn to use the toilet, but she will be made miserable in the process (and so will her parents). In extreme cases, certain types of misguided "training" are likely to impede this learning or produce in the child a refusal to defecate, which will result in constipation.

Yet how will she learn if we never take her nappy off? Will she wear a nappy for the rest of her life? I doubt it. I don't know anyone who has tried it, but I suspect that even if their parents did nothing, children would end up taking their nappy off themselves. No one wears a nappy aged fifteen. But the fact is that nappies are expensive and changing them requires an effort and, sooner or later, almost all parents try to wean their children off wearing nappies.

In theory, this shouldn't be a problem. Nappies are completely artificial; a relatively recent invention, designed for the comfort of parents, not children. Children don't need nappies. Many parents take off their child's nappy in the summer, leaving things to chance. Sometimes they do this before the child is a year old, even though they know it is impossible for them to control their bodily functions. It is of course preferable not to have rugs or carpets in the house when you do this, and you need to be ready to mop up anywhere at a moment's notice without getting cross. That way the child is spared nappy rash for a while, and the parents save a lot of money. If the child is still not dry when summer is over, the nappies go back on and everyone is happy.

The first summer after she is two, when there is a real possibility of development, the parents can explain to their child what they expect of her: "When you want to do a pee or a poo, tell mummy or daddy." Needless to say, there is no need to pester her every half hour (it is enough to explain once in June or at most every fortnight), and she shouldn't be put on her potty, unless she asks to be, or told off, or criticised or laughed at if she has an accident or a false alarm, nor should you lose your patience. It might be useful to ask her if she prefers to use the toilet, like mummy and daddy, or a potty, or a child's toilet seat (and to choose the one she likes most). Unless she has a minimum of control, it is advisable to put a nappy on her when you go out.

Some children will start to control themselves that summer, others the summer after. For some this will occur naturally before or after, and they will ask to stop wearing nappies in the winter ("Are you sure?" "Yes." "All right, let's give it a try.").

As I said, stopping using nappies shouldn't be a problem, but it can be. Even without you forcing them, telling them off, pestering them, or making offensive comments, some children simply refuse to stop wearing nappies. They are so accustomed to wearing them they can't imagine life without them. Explain to your child that it doesn't matter where she does a pee or a poo, you won't be angry. But if, in spite of everything, she asks to wear a nappy, put it on her without saying a word. After all, the nappy wasn't her idea; her parents were the ones who decided she should wear them when she was born and it isn't the poor little girl's fault if she has got used to them. A child who was happy for you to take her nappy off at one and a half may refuse at two and a half. Don't insist, don't pester her, just say: "All right, when you want to take it off, tell mummy or daddy."

Some children are quite content not to wear a nappy, but feel unable to sit on a potty. They want to go, they tell you so, but refuse to sit anywhere. They want a nappy. Sometimes, you have to put a nappy on them every time they want to do a pee or a poo. Some children, who run around naked on the beach, need to have a nappy put on in order to do a pee. Don't be surprised, don't complain, don't laugh at them. Put the nappy on without arguing, it won't be long now. Some children, who are more timid, won't dare to ask for a nappy, but they won't use a potty, so they try to hold on as long as possible. Some even become constipated. If you notice your child stops doing a poo when you take her nappy off, offer to put it back on (even if she doesn't ask).

There is nothing wrong with going back to using nappies after a few days or months of stopping using them. It isn't a step backwards or a regression, and it won't do your child any harm. Unless, of course, she doesn't want it.

Now let's look at the other extreme, at the child who is unable to control her bodily functions, but who refuses to wear a nappy, or who won't go back to wearing one after the summer. As always, it is essential to speak to the child and to be respectful. If she only has occasional accidents, then it is best to do what she wants. If she has no control at all, you might be able to persuade her to wear it. But if she absolutely refuses, if she cries when you try to put it on and experiences it as a failure or a disgrace, it is also best to do as she wants, perhaps to try to reach a compromise ("You can stop wearing a nappy at home but you have to wear one if we go out for a walk."). There will be times when you have to sacrifice going out for a few weeks in order to avoid a drama, which is a bore. To prevent this, it is important not to make heavy weather of it, not to drop hints or make hurtful remarks, or for anyone to say to the poor child, "What a disgrace, a big girl like you wearing a nappy", "When are you going to learn to use the toilet", "If you wet yourself again, I'll put you in nappies again, like a baby", and other choice remarks. One must never speak to a child in this way, about this or any other matter.

For the past few years, some parents have decided not to put their children in nappies from the beginning, thus avoiding the problem of having to stop using them (as well as the financial and environmental cost). This isn't such a crazy idea; obviously humans lived for many years without nappies, and even today the majority of children in the world still don't use them. Of course, this doesn't mean potty-training a child, or shouting at or threatening her if she soils herself; it means paying great attention in order (for us) to learn to know when she is about to go, and to accept without complaining if she goes when we are unprepared. Because my children were too grown up when I found out about this, I wasn't able to try it out and therefore have no first-hand experience. Books have been written on the subject, although as far as I know none have been published in Spain. You can find information on the Internet.[91]

Every normal child will be able to control herself during the day, without being taught. If your child continues to pee or poo in her pants over the age of four (apart from wetting herself occasionally), go to see a paediatrician.

When problems exist, they are often psychological (these can sometimes be due to forced potty training, or they can be a sign of other conflicts, or of jealousy). In some cases, involuntary soiling (encopresis) is a result of constipation: a ball is formed that irritates the rectal mucosa producing "false diarrhea". The child doesn't do this on purpose, and ridicule and punishment will only make the problem worse.

However, night-time is a very different matter. Although many children are dry at night by the age of three, many others wet the bed (nocturnal enuresis) until they become teenagers and sometimes throughout their lives. During World War I (1914–18), 1 percent of American soldiers were disqualified from military service due to enuresis. Night enuresis almost never has a physical or psychological cause, but depends more on neurological development and is genetically determined (it is hereditary).

Some children manage not to wet the bed on special occasions (for example, at a friend's house), at the cost of staying awake almost the whole night. Obviously, they can't keep this up for days at a time. Unfortunately, some parents are unaware of the huge effort involved, and reproach the child ("You made an effort at Pablo's house, but here at home you don't care – of course, you've got me to wash your sheets."). This type of remark is not only cruel, it is untrue. A mother recently wrote on an Internet forum that her seven-year-old daughter wets the bed. Another mother posted the following response:

> *I wet the bed until I was seventeen, and I felt dreadful and had a terrible inferiority complex... I used to stay awake for hours at night so as not to wet the bed, and would wet myself during the five minutes when I nodded off; I wouldn't have anything to drink after twelve o'clock, it was awful, and I kept on wetting myself; I used to get up at night to wash the sheets so no one would find out... Don't tell her off, don't make her feel guilty, it's an illness, and then one day it stopped. My eldest son wet the bed until he was thirteen...*

I would like to tell a story here, in honour of a great Japanese paediatrician, Dr Itsuro Yamanouchi, from Okayama. I visited his hospital once in 1988, and was fascinated by this modest, wise man, who, despite being the head of a big hospital, continued seeing patients at his surgery. One afternoon I went along to be present at one of his consultations, and he explained to me in English what the problem was:

"This boy is six, and he wets his bed. I told his mother this is normal, he doesn't need any treatment, and that I wet my bed until I was seven."

"What a coincidence, so did I!", I replied in my hesitant English.

Much to my surprise, Dr Yamanouchi quickly translated what I had said, and the mother looked at me in astonishment, and began bowing and thanking me profusely.

A while later, another mother, when hearing the doctor's words, also looked at me in astonishment and bowed.

"This child is ten and he wets his bed, too. I explained to his mother I wet my bed until I was eleven, and that you did until you were seven."

"But… didn't you say you wet yours until you were seven?"

"Well", Dr Yamanouchi grinned, "I always add on a year."

Look, but don't touch

The Sunday supplement of *El Periodico* contains a section devoted to laughing at celebrities. On page 4 of the October 17 1999 edition, there is an article entitled "Child attached", in which a journalist was poking fun at people who have been photographed carrying their child:

> Many celebrities have decided to park their designer prams at home and carry their sprogs themselves. This regression to Neolithic methods may be of some educational value, but it can't be very healthy or comfortable.

The resourceful journalist seems to think the pram was invented at the end of the Neolithic period, and that no one has carried a child since. Have you noticed any Bronze Age, Greek, Roman, Assyrian, Medieval, Renaissance or Baroque prams in museums lately? No. Prams are a relatively new invention, and up until very recently people carried their children.

> However little your child weighs, carrying him will take its toll in the form of a twisted spine or a discal hernia.

This is arrant nonsense. Carrying a child won't cause a twisted spine or a discal hernia.

Moreover, it is arguable whether a child prefers hanging like an appendage or lying on his back in a nice soft pram.

We can argue about it if you like. However, a child crying his eyes out in a pram, who calms down as soon as he is picked up appears to know exactly what he prefers.

Riding along in rhythm to mummy or daddy's steps may be stimulating, but it is also tiring.

I am prepared to admit it may be tiring for a parent to carry a child, especially if he is plump. But how can it be tiring for the child? When you pay attention to your child, and give him what he wants (a feed, to be carried or allowed to sleep in your bed), it is quite common for people even to accuse you of harming him.

In any event, carrying your child around like Cindy Crawford does, as if he were a parcel, seems very unwise, more than anything because babies need to breathe.

As if he were a parcel? In the photo, the model is carrying her baby lovingly in a comfortable sling. This method is very sensible, because it is safe, it distributes the baby's weight evenly, and allows the mother to move her arms relatively freely. And, of course, the baby is able to breathe perfectly well. Isn't it more likely the jealous journalist would be out of breath if only he could get that close to Cindy!

In contrast, Antonio David Flores is carrying his daughter too loosely. She rests on his shoulder, disdainfully, like one leaning on the counter in a bar.

The image that produced such an acerbic response is of a little girl of three or four looking as happy as anything in the arms of her daddy. I can't see anything disdainful in the way she is resting on his shoulder. Sometimes, the disdain is in the eyes of the beholder...

The article is simply an example of the prejudice against carrying children that is rife in our society. Yes, of course, the article is frivolous, a mere joke, and yet what parents haven't had to listen to similar remarks from relatives, friends, even strangers?

Some time ago a title in a bookshop caught my eye: *Hug Me, Mummy.*[32] It looked promising. A book clearly in favour of contact between mother and child! But no, it is the same old idea of "freedom within limits". True, the author can't praise physical contact enough, attributing to it properties that had never even occurred to me: "It stimulates [the child's] brain", "it is a form of communication", "it transmits affection", "the child feels your heart beating and this calms him":

> The psychological benefits of physical contact at that age are undeniable. It has been proven that if during the first year of life a child is deprived of physical contact, or the rocking movement he experiences when carried in a sling, he will have difficulty making social contact with other children and as an adult will display aggressive behaviour.

I can scarcely believe that carrying a child can be that important. If all this is true, we should go and pick up our children immediately, right? But be careful, there are some exceptions. *Hug Me, Mummy* suggests that it is inadvisable to pick him up:

- If you are anxious, because you will certainly pass on your anxiety to him.
- In order to quieten him.

- So that he goes to sleep.
- When… you can't take anymore!
- If he refuses to walk.

In short: pick up your child at any time, except when he needs it and when you need it. If you are that mother in the advertisement, running in slow motion, barefoot, dressed in dazzling white, through a green field, blonde hair billowing in the breeze (and without treading on any nettles), and beside you two flaxen-haired, impeccably-behaved children (who never squabble!) are playing with a golden retriever whose coat also billows in the breeze, then you may hold your plump, smiling baby, who doesn't pee or poo or have a runny nose, and transmit your affection to him, stimulate his brain and let him smell the cleanness of your clothes.

However, if you are a confused first-time mother (or if you have to alternate looking after your baby with attending to a jealous sibling or two unruly siblings), if since you gave birth there are days when you burst into tears for no reason, if you have reproached your husband for not helping enough and he has stormed out, if your mother and your mother-in-law have come "to help out" and criticise everything you do, if no one has come to help and the dirty dishes and the ironing are piling up and you haven't been able to sleep a wink, then don't be so selfish as to go and pick up your baby, smother him with kisses, sit down with him and forget all your cares. No! You are anxious and you might pass your anxiety on to him! Why not buy a lottery ticket instead and win the jackpot, then you can hire a couple of servants and a nanny and come back when you are feeling more relaxed. If you hurry up, you might get to hold him before he finishes primary school.

Are you aware of any quicker way to stop a baby from crying or to send him to sleep than by picking him up and singing to him? They say gas works more quickly, but I have never tried it, and of course I wouldn't recommend it. And if your one-and-a-half-year-old child refuses to walk and it is time to go home, what choice do you have but to pick him up? Will you wait until he feels like walking, even if you have to go to sleep on a bench next to the sand pit? Will you drag him through the streets by his hair?

It seems deliberately obstructive: like saying, "Water is very good for you, but you must never drink it when you are thirsty, or "You sleep more soundly in a bed, but you must never fall asleep in one."

Time-out!

Time-out, or exclusion, is one of the "educational" techniques derived from Behaviourism. One of its advocates is Dr Christophersen, Professor of Paediatrics and Science at Kansas University. He published a lengthy exposé of his methods in a prestigious paediatric journal.[83] It is true that at first sight they seem fairly common-sensical; he firmly rejects corporal punishment, and goes on to explain that children under four or five aren't capable of abstract thought, and therefore can't carry out many of our commands. He also points out that children learn through repetition, so that when they do something "badly" again and again, they aren't being naughty or disobedient, they are simply practising. He argues that the exclusion method "works much better than spanking, yelling, and threatening children", which no doubt is also true...

Yet when you read the detailed description of the method, you wonder where all the common sense went. We are speaking of children of between eight months and twelve years old, who have done things such as "tantrums, hitting and other aggressive acts, failure to follow directions [...] jumping on furniture, and interrupting". The procedure is as follows:

Step 1. Following the inappropiate behavior, say to your child,

"No, don't _____". Say this calmly, without raising your voice, talking angrily, or nagging. Carry her to the playpen without saying another word, with her facing away from you so she does not mistake it for affection.

Step 2: After she is in the playpen, do not say a word, do not look at her, and do not talk about her. After she has stopped crying and is relaxed, go to the playpen, pick her up without saying a word and set her on the floor near some of her toys. Do not reprimand her or mention what she did wrong. You do not need to lecture her and should try not to be angry. If she begins crying when you walk toward her or as you pick her up, place her back in the playpen and start over.

Step 3. After each time-out, children should start out with a "clean slate." No discussion, no nagging, threatening or reminding is necessary. At the first opportunity, look for and praise positive behaviors.

The child can be punished at any moment, without prior warning, for an unlimited time, by an all-powerful being, who offers no explanation and pretends not to be angry. The accused can say nothing in his defence, because the decision is irreversible.

The only way a child can put an end to the sentence is by stopping crying. And promising not to do it again won't help if he is still crying when he makes that promise. Being excluded for a prescribed length of time isn't enough: a convicted murderer will get out of prison after eighteen years, whether he cries or not, whether he repents or not, whether he apologises or not; but an excluded child may remain there indefinitely if he doesn't stop crying (fortunately, parents usually have more common sense than "experts", and if a child doesn't calm down after a reasonable length of time, they will end up picking him up). The child is being asked to repress his feelings and to stop crying precisely when he has the strongest urge (and reason) to do so. He is being asked to pretend (and to lie to himself), to repress his own personality and transform himself into a robot so as to satisfy his parents' wishes. It would be difficult to conceive of a more inhumane method.

Why shouldn't parents raise their voice to the child or nag him? In order to show him they are superior; this is about not stooping to his level, about showing him you have the self-assuredness and composure of a god incarnate.

Why this insistence on not talking to or looking at the child? Because people understand each other through talking, and for the Behaviourist it is essential that parent and child don't communicate. If they do, the child may argue, defend, plead, challenge and the process may be contaminated by an element of reason. The ability to talk is what distinguishes man from the animals; and, let us not forget, Skinner experimented with rats. If you look at your child, you may see his suffering, you may feel compassion, you may make eye contact. All of these things endanger the success of the method, which on principle must be distant, impersonal, irrational and merciless.

Why must the child not mistake the procedure for affection? Because picking up a child and placing him in the playpen is the method's weak point: in environments where picking up children is strictly prohibited because it "spoils" them, the poor wretched child might think that by picking him up we are showing him affection. He may "misbehave" on purpose, so that his parents touch or speak to him.

Within certain limits, children suffer more from their parents' indifference than from being shouted at or hit. Using indifference may seem like progress, more "humane" than shouting or lecturing, but it is simply a regression towards a more exquisite form of torture. Indifference, like electric shocks, is the perfect torture: it is more painful than a beating, but leaves no physical mark.

Why during the time-out must parents not mention to the child what he has done wrong? Wouldn't verbal reinforcement make the method more effective? ("Don't touch the gas knobs, don't hit your little brother.") God forbid! Explaining only weakens the effect. The accused might deny the facts, or even (in a supreme act of defiance!) the validity of the rule. A regime of terror can't allow any debate.

Why does the method only apply to the under-twelves? Wouldn't it be a good way of modifying the behaviour of, say, a sarcastic student, an idle worker, a rude customer, an insensitive boyfriend, a disobedient wife? No, and there are three reasons why not. Firstly, a child over twelve is too heavy to pick up and put in a playpen. Secondly, he won't keep quiet when treated with such an obvious lack of respect. Thirdly, and perhaps most importantly, it would be embarrassing: the mere idea of subjecting a teenager or an adult to that kind of humiliation would cause amazement, laughter or concern. And yet it seems so "normal" to treat a child that way…

(Incidentally, dear reader, did the expression "disobedient wife" in the previous paragraph bother you? It is shocking isn't it? We refer now to this kind of language as "sexist" – the worst type of politically incorrect language. Why, then, is it acceptable to say "disobedient child"?)

A few readers will have had a feeling of *déjà vu* on reading the explanations of the time-out method. Where have you read something similar before? Here perhaps:

"You can't leave, you're under arrest."

"So it seems," said K. "But why?" he asked.

"We're not at liberty to say. Go back to your room and wait there. […]"

"You're under arrest."

"But, how can I just be under arrest like that?"

"There you go again," said the guard, dipping a morsel of bread into the honey jar. "We don't answer that sort of question."

"Well you should. Here are my papers, now show me yours, but firstly I want to see an arrest warrant."

"Heavens!" said the guard. "You can't accept your situation, and you seem to want to irritate us for no reason."

These passages are from Kafka's *The Trial* (1925). Yes, the time-out method is Kafkaesque in the strictest sense of the word.

But is it successful? Almost all of the methods I take issue with in this book are. They succeed in their aim: to produce a submissive, obedient child, who is no trouble. The problem is whether we agree with that aim or not, whether blind obedience and respectful silence are the qualities we most wish to nurture in our child.

Yet it doesn't succeed completely, of course; as Christophersen himself unwittingly and ingenuously admits when he explains to us the written rules distributed to parents of children (under eighteen months) at nurseries in the greater metropolitan area of Kansas. There are a few positive points among them: members of staff are forbidden to smack or shout at the children. (How ironical! Here we have a champion of the time-out method converted into what Dr Green refers to as an "anti-corporal punishment lobbyist".) But this is where genuine discipline comes into play:

> If a child exhibits an unacceptable behavior, the nearest available staff person will issue a brief verbal statement, "no," proceed to the child, pick him/her up securely but not forcefully, transport him/her to the playpen, and gently place him/her in it. As soon as he/she is relaxed and quiet, a staff person will remove him/her from the playpen and return him/her to an appropriate area.

If the unacceptable behaviour "places other children at risk" and continues after the time-out,

> [...] the child will be disenrolled from the Center, and the parents requested to locate another placement for their child.

The result couldn't be more perfect:

[...] the overall day-care atmosphere improved dramatically after the one or two problem children either improved their behavior or were disenrolled.

When we speak of "placing other children at risk", we think of teenagers taking their father's assault rifle and firing at fellow pupils in the playground. Yet if we reflect about the ability of a child under eighteen months to be aggressive, in an enclosed space supervised by adults, we can only conclude that the "risk" posed to other children is the possibility of having their dummy snatched or being pushed and falling onto their backsides (padded with nappies). Failing all attempts to solve these serious problems, the learned Behaviourists from Kansas have been obliged to expel these renegade babies from the nurseries. Will they be sent to reform-nurseries, or will they join dangerous street gangs of delinquent babies? Can you imagine the life of crime that might await a child who is expelled for bad behaviour at fourteen months old? Sadly, this is no joke. What idea will parents have of their child when they are told he has been expelled for "untreatable unacceptable behavior"? ("Look, Madam, we have no choice but to expel your fourteen-month-old child. He shows aggressive behaviour that endangers other children, and the most advanced treatments in modern psychology have proved hopeless in his case. We can do nothing more to help him. Buy a gun, and may God protect you.") What will they say at the next nursery or school you take your child to? ("It says here he was expelled from his last nursery. On what grounds?"). If this is the best the system can do to help "problem" babies, what sort of disciplinary measures will it take with children aged five, seven or thirteen?

Expelling a fourteen-month-old child from a nursery because of unacceptable or uncontrollable behaviour is a tragic admission of incompetence. Others, who haven't as many university degrees, have devoted more time to looking and talking to children. I remember, for example, that at our first son's nursery, there was a boy who used to bite the other children. "We have to be very patient with him," said Estela and Gloria, two excellent child carers, "there are problems at home. But with love and patience, he will stop biting." And of course he stopped.

In order to highlight the attributes of his method, Christophersen can't resist adding a "humane" touch:

> [...] many children who have been raised using time-out will place their dolls and their peers in time-out for misbehavior. [...] children who are spanked by their parents will spank their dolls and their peers, and children who are constantly verbally reprimanded will reprimand their dolls and their peers similarly.

No, let us not be afraid to finish the sentence: : *and those who are treated with constant affection and respect do the same to their dolls and peers.*

It is sad that someone can come so close to the truth without seeing it. Indeed, toddlers don't hit their fellow children because they "haven't been properly brought up", they hit them because they have been "brought up" by parents who hit them. And the time-out method isn't the solution, because even though it stops the child from hitting, it doesn't teach him to treat his friends with affection, only to "exclude" them.

Early stimulation

There are some excellent professionals devoted to the care of children with disabilities, and I am sure that early stimulation may be very useful in such cases.

The myth I want to debunk here is that early stimulation of healthy children can produce geniuses.[84]

As myths go this can be a fairly innocuous one if it merely

leads to parents spending more time with their child, playing with her, teaching her songs and reading her stories. All of this, of course, is good for children.

However, the ends (increased intelligence) may render the means unjustifiable. Let us assume, for example, that children learn to speak earlier if their parents play with them and read them stories. Will this appear on their CV? ("At what age did you begin to speak?" "I said 'daddy' at eleven months, and at eighteen months I had a vocabulary of eighty-five words." "Wonderful, the job is yours.") Being able to demonstrate that a child is slightly ahead at aged two obviously isn't enough, there must still be a difference when she is twenty-five for any long-term effect to be proven.

And if there were any long-term effect, what exactly would have been the key to this success? The games, the stories, the songs? What provides more stimulus, "The Three Little Pigs" or hide-n-seek? Or did those parents also send their children to the best schools, or help them more with their homework when they were twelve? Don't parents who devote more time to their children when they are very young continue to do so for the rest of their lives?

"Play with your child in order to enjoy these years" sounds like good advice for young parents. Saying, "Stimulate your child so she becomes more intelligent" doesn't. Children's games aren't competitive, nobody wins at peek-a-boo or loses at tickling. Yet with stimulation there can be a loser, because there is an objective (intelligence). Parents play in order to laugh and to enjoy seeing their children laugh, but stimulation can be turned into an obligation for both children and parents, who may think they have the right to receive something in exchange for their "efforts". ("Be quiet, I tell you, don't interrupt when I'm telling you a story!" "What do you mean 'what's a palace?' I explained to you what a palace is yesterday. You should pay more attention.") What parents convey to their child when they play with her isn't knowledge or learning skills, but rather the wonderful feeling of being loved and respected, of being important.

One of the greatest dangers of this myth is the widely held belief that parents don't know how to stimulate their children properly, and that this is the job of experts in pedagogy. Parents are made to believe their child needs to go to the nursery in order to learn how to talk, to become socialised (i.e. to be able to relate to other children), to "sharpen their wits" in general, to be less spoiled, to be separated from their mothers (this the nurseries acomplish, unfortunately: to separate children from their mothers).

This is untrue. Going to a nursery is not better for a child than being at home with her family. In 1991, Susan Dilks carried out an in-depth review of scientific studies comparing children who went to nursery school with those who stayed at home with their parents.[85] Attending a nursery school was associated with a less stable emotional bond with parents. As for socialisation, the data was conflicting: some studies showed a higher degree of socialisation, but others showed more aggression; the results were better in the high quality nursery schools. In terms of learning and intelligence there was no difference between children who went to nursery school and those who stayed at home, except among children from poorer backgrounds, who showed some improvement if they attended high quality nursery schools attached to departments of pedagogical science at universities. Any improvements in learning disappeared unless those children received special support throughout their schooling. Nothing was said about children from wonderful families (like your own, dear reader) who attend poor quality nursery schools.

In 2007, Bradley and Vandell encountered a similar overall situation:[93] children who attended nursery school had more developed language skills, especially children from poor backgrounds who attended high quality nursery schools; but they also had behavioural problems, were aggressive and suffered from stress, especially those who had started nursery school younger, and had attended for more hours during the day.

To conclude, if a child receives proper treatment at home, attending nursery school won't give her any advantages.

Of course, thousands of families have to send their children to nursery school for economic reasons. While we are struggling to extend maternity leave, it is good to know that a child can develop more or less as well in a high quality nursery school as at home.

And how do we tell these high quality nursery schools we keep talking about apart? Dilks offers a series of general criteria, for example regarding the number of children per carer: a maximum of four children under eighteen months old, or five children between eighteen and thirty-six months old, or eight children between three and five years old. The American Academy of Paediatrics recommends even more stringent figures:[94] A maximum of three children under one year old, or four between thirteen and thirty months old, or five between thirty-one and thirty-five months old, or seven three-year-olds, or eight four- or five-year-olds. How many children are there per carer in your nursery school?

Spanish legislation permits eight children of under one year old per carer. Do you think it is possible to look after eight babies at once? If you had octuplets, or even quadruplets, would you feel able to look after them all day with no one to help you? You would spend the whole time feeding them and changing their nappies; it would be impossible to do anything else with them. Where would the famous early stimulation come into play, or just simple affection? Who do you think plays with your child or picks her up when she cries? How can you be surprised that when you collect her in the afternoon, she wants to be cuddled all the time?

The problem is that childcare has been designed along purely economic lines. The criteria hasn't been: "Children's needs are these, and the cost will be this much, so let's see where we can get the money from", but rather quite the opposite: "We have this much money, let's see what we can achieve with it." And the amount of money available is, by definition, very small, because the mother can't spend more than a certain part of what she earns on childcare, and in general women are paid less than men.

And so, the whole of our education system is topsy-turvy. The younger the pupil, the less experience and qualifications their teachers are expected to have, and the lower their salary. Arguably, it should be the other way round: nursery carers should be better qualified and better paid than university teachers, because a baby can suffer greatly at the hands of a bad carer, while a twenty-year-old youth couldn't care less about a bad physics teacher.

In general, the hourly rate paid to baby-sitters is lower than that paid to cleaners. Which is more important, that your child is well cared for, or that the floors are polished?

Because it is so badly paid, childcare is looked down upon. And on top of that, when a mother makes a huge economic sacrifice by stopping working for a few months in order to look after her baby, people say, "You're lucky to be able to afford to" or, "Lucky you, all day with nothing to do", or even, "Don't give up your career, you'll vegetate…" A while ago, I read a comment from a mother, who, fed up with being criticised, had decided that instead of saying, "I'm not working at the moment", she would say: "I'm taking part in a research project in applied psychology to study the effects of prolonged one-to-one contact on the psychoemotional development of babies."

It sounded so complicated that nobody dared ask for more details, and so they didn't realise she was the researcher, her study subject was her child, the study centre her house, and that she wasn't being paid for her work.

Quality time

Their parents are suffered to see them only
twice a year; the visit is to last but an hour . . .
Jonathan Swift, GULLIVER'S TRAVELS

Many parents are clear that nursery school isn't the best solution, and they only resort to it because they are forced by necessity. Rather than going to the root of the problem, and creating social and economical conditions that would enable each family to choose freely, many people have chosen to make a leap of faith: to sing the praises of nursery school and assure mothers there is no problem.

Mothers are told that, even though they are separated from their child for eight hours a day (which, including travel, can easily become ten), they can care for him equally well, because it is quality not quantity that matters. And in two hours of "quality time" they can do as much as other mothers do in ten or twelve.

I confess that the idea seemed more or less acceptable to me, until I had to experience it at first hand, when as a paediatrician I asked for paternal leave in order to spend more time with my children. You give up your work, your salary, any hope of promotion or a raise, the social plaudits of a professional career. As nursery schools are heavily funded, your family, with only one wage earner, has to pay taxes to help subsidize the nursery school for children whose parents both work. And on top of all that you have to listen to remarks such as: "Well, I don't see the point of you being at home. I spend less time with my son, but what matters is that it's quality time."

And who says my time isn't quality time? The time my children and I spend together is of equal quality and there is more of it.

We should try convincing our employers of this: "From now

on, I will only come to work for two hours, but since this will be quality time, I will do the same amount of work as others do in eight hours and I'll earn the same amount." It doesn't wash, does it? In any job or activity, from bricklaying to piano playing, you will only succeed by investing time. Why is caring for our children the only human activity where time becomes flexible?

EPILOGUE
The happiest day

My hearth is touched now, by many remembrances that had long fallen asleep, of my pretty young mother (and I so old!)
Charles Dickens, A TALE OF TWO CITIES

As children, almost all of us have written a school essay entitled "The happiest day of my life". In religious schools you were assured of success if you wrote about your first communion. Others preferred recalling the biggest, most expensive Christmas present Santa Claus had brought them, a trip to a far away country, a visit to the funfair…

As the years go by our outlook changes, objects fade and people take on an unexpected importance. Our mother's smile, our father's embrace, a friend's hand in ours, a word of encouragement, or thanks, or forgiveness… Search your memory, dear reader. What were the happiest days of your childhood?

This is how Manuel describes one of those indelible memories:

I must have been about six or seven. I was running through the house, which was dark, and I collided with a glass door that was normally open. The glass shattered and fell around my feet. I got a big shock, and a tiny cut on my forehead. Yet I felt no pain: I was paralysed with fear of being punished. My father came running, extracted me from the pile of glass, treated my cut, and examined me from head to toe. But he didn't scold me. To begin with, I was shaking, expecting at any moment to hear a dreadful roar. Then I thought he had forgotten to scold me, and I tried to make myself small. But finally, my surprise and curiosity got the better of me, and, still tearful, I asked him: "Aren't you angry with me for breaking the door?" "No", he replied, "the door doesn't matter, all that matters to me is that you didn't hurt yourself." I understand now that as parents we all value our children more than anything in the world. Yet we rarely say this to our children. I am very grateful to my father for having said it to me.

This is Encarna's story:

One of the happiest days I remember actually began rather badly. I had a horrible nightmare. Not about monsters or bogeymen, but about an oyster, an enormous oyster pushing an equally enormous pearl out of its shell, and not allowing it back in again. I felt terribly sorry for the poor ejected pearl. I woke up screaming, truly terrified. I must have been about five at the time, and I used to sleep in a cot next to my parents' bed. They, of course, woke up, alarmed by my screams. My mother invited me into her bed to sleep. All my fears vanished as if by magic, and I felt incredibly happy and safe. I never had another nightmare. I knew I would always have a refuge, that someone would always protect me.

I, for my part, recall one afternoon, I think it was a Sunday, when I was twelve. I was mooching round the house, bored. My mother caught hold of me, and said: "Come and sit on my lap, like when you were little". I imagine I must have died of embarrassment, yet I don't remember being embarrased. What I do remember, on the other hand, is that she began singing very softly:

Rockabye baby on the tree top
When the wind blows the cradle will rock…

I leaned my head on her breast, and was filled with a sensation of infinite calm. I almost fell asleep. It was like being two years old again.

Most people have no memory of being a baby. I know what a baby feels in its mother's arms because I had the enormous good fortune to be a baby again for half an hour when I was twelve years old.

All of these stories have something in common. The happiest moments of our childhood are those in which our parents (or grandparents, or brothers and sisters, or friends) made us happy. Even when we think what made us happy was an electric train set, if we look more closely people are behind everything: our parents who gave it to us with a smile, or a word of praise, a brother with whom (not always willingly) we shared our train set...

We were children and now we are parents. Many years have gone by, and yet so little time that the change of role sometimes surprises us. Suddenly we see our own childhood and our own parents in a different light. We look at our children and we wonder which day, which words, which adventure will remain etched in their memory; which suffering will be lodged in their hearts, and which joys they will treasure.

The happiest days of your child's life are yet to come. They depend on you.

References

1. GARCÍA, P. A., *Compendio de pedagogía teórico-práctica*. Librería de Perlado, Páez y compañía, Madrid, 1909.
2. LANGIS, R., *Aprende a decir "NO" a tus hijos*. Editorial Sirio, Málaga, 1999.
3. GRAY, C., Pediatricians taking a new look at the corporal-punishment issue. *CMAJ* 2002, 19; 166:793. http://www.cmaj.ca/cgi/content/full/166/6/793?
4. MIRANDA BELLO, J., *Vida y color 2*. Álbumes Españoles, Barcelona, 1968.
5. TAYLOR, S. E., *The Tending Instinct*. Henry Holt & Co, 2002.
6. NELSON, E. A. S., SCHIEFENHOEVEL, S. and HAIMERL, F., Child care practices in nonindustrialized societies. *Pediatrics*, 2000, 105. http://www.pediatrics.org/cgi/content/full/105/6/e75.pdf
7. ALLPORT, S., *A Natural History of Parenting*. Harmony Books, New York, 1997.
8. KOI, S., *Family and Orphan Rabbit Care*. The Kind Planet, http://www.kindplanet.org/rabbitbabies.html
9. LEBAS, F., COUDERT, P., ROUVIER, R. and ROCHAMBEAU, H. de, *Rabbit Husbandry, Health and Production*. FAO, Rome, 1986. http://www.fao.org/docrep/x5082e/X5082E07.htm
10. LAWRENCE, R. A. and LAWRENCE, R. M., *Breastfeeding, a Guide for the Medical Profession*. 5.ª ed. Mosby, St. Louis, 1999.
11. BOWLBY, J., *Attachment*. Pimlico, 1997.
12. PUIG and ROIG, P., *Puericultura*. Librería Subirana, Barcelona, 1927.
13. KRAMER, M. S., CHALMERS, B., HODNETT, E. D., SEVKOVSKAYA, Z., DZIKOVICH, I., SHAPIRO, S., et ál., Promotion of breastfeeding intervention trial (PROBIT). A randomized trial in the Republic of Belarus. *JAMA*, 2001, 285:413-420.
14. CHRISTENSSON, K., SILES, C., MORENO, L., BELAUSTEQUI, A., FUENTE, P. DE LA, LAGERCRANTZ, H., PUYOL, P. and WINBERG, J., Temperature, metabolic adaptation and crying in healthy fullterm newborns cared for skin-to-skin or in a cot. *Acta Paediatr.*, 1992, 81: 488–493.
15. ESTIVILL, E. and BÉJAR, S. DE, *Duérmete, niño*. 2.ª ed. Plaza & Janés,

Barcelona, 1996.

16. BOWLBY, J., *Child Care and the Growth of Love.* 2.ª ed. Penguin Books, London, 1990.

17. FERBER, R., *Solve Your Child's Sleep Problems.* Dorling Kindersley, London, 1986.

18. CYRULNIK, B., *Los patitos feos.* Gedisa, Barcelona, 2002.

19. MORELLI, G. A., ROGOFF, B., OPPENHEIM, D. and GOLDSMITH, D., Cultural variation in infants sleeping arrangements: questions of independence. *Dev. Psychol.,* 1992, 28:604–613.

20. SMALL, M. F., *Our Babies, Ourselves.* Anchor Books, New York, 1999.

21. ELIAS, M. F., NICOLSON, N. A., BORA, C. and JOHNSTON, J., Sleep/wake patterns of breast-fed infants in the first 2 years of life. *Pediatrics,* 1986, 77:322–329.

22. STUART-MACADAM, P. and DETTWYLER, K. A., *Breastfeeding, Biocultural Perspectives.* Aldine de Gruyter, New York, 1995.

23. SUGARMAN, M. and KENDALL-TACKETT, K., Weaning ages in a sample of American women who practice extended breastfeeding. *Clinical Pediatrics,* 1995; 34:642–647.

24. JACKSON, D., *Three in a Bed, the Benefits of Sleeping with Your Baby.* Bloomsbury Publishing, London, 1999.

25. THEVENIN ,T., *The Family Bed.* Avery Publishing Group, Wayne, New Jersey, 1987.

26. SEARS,W., *Nighttime Parenting. How to Get Your Baby and Child to Sleep.* La Leche League International, Schaumburg, Illinois, 1999.

27. SAMPEDRO, J. L., *La sonrisa etrusca.* Alfaguara, Madrid, 1992.

28. KESELMAN, G. and VILLAMUZA, N., *De verdad que no podía.* Editorial Kókinos, Madrid, 2002. http://www.editorialkokinos.com/cuentos/deverdad.html

29. BLAIR, P. S., FLEMING, P. J., SMITH, I. J., PLATT, M. W., YOUNG, J., NADIN, P., BERRY, P. J., GOLDING, J., the CESDI SUDI RESEARCH GROUP, Babies sleeping with parents: case-control study of factors influencing the risk of the sudden infant death syndrome. *Br. Med. J.,* 1999, 319:1457-1462.

30. MURRAY, L., FIORI-COWLEY, A., HOOPER, R. and COOPER, P., The impact of postnatal depression and associated adversity on early mother-infant interactions and later infant outcome. *Child. Dev.,* 1996 Oct.; 67(5):2512-2526.

31. BOWLBY, J., *A Secure Base*. Basic Books, New York, 1988.
32. FERRERÓS TOR, M. L., *Abrázame, mamá*. Tibidabo Ediciones, Barcelona, 1999.
33. STIRNIMANN, F., *El niño*. Seix Barral, Barcelona, 1947.
34. SKINNER, B. F., *Walden Two*. Hackett Publishing Co, 2005.
35. MILLER, A., *For Your Own Good: Roots of Violence in Child-rearing*. Virago Press, 1987.
36. KOLLER, T. and WILLI, H., *La madre y el niño*. 2.ª ed. Delfos, Barcelona, 1946.
37. RAMOS, R., *Puericultura*. Barcelona, Autoedición, 1941.
38. BOWLBY, J., *La separación afectiva*. Paidós, Barcelona, 1993.
39. CLOSA MONASTEROLO, R., MORALEJO BENÉITEZ, J., RAVÉS OLIVÉ, M. M., MARTÍNEZ MARTÍNEZ, M. J. and GÓMEZ PAPÍ, A., Método canguro en recién nacidos prematuros ingresados en una Unidad de Cuidados Intensivos Neonatal. *An. Esp. Pediatr.*, 1998, 49:495–498.
40. VARGAS, JULIE S., *Brief Biography of B.F. Skinner*. http://www.bfskinner.org/BFSkinner/AboutSkinner.html
41. Kibbutz Ketura, Children. http://www.ketura.org.il/child.html
42. LOTHANE, Z., Daniel Paul Schreber, the most famous patient in psychiatry and psychoanalysis. http://www.mssm.edu/faculty/lothane/schreber/histo.html
43. MORTON SCHATZMAN, Another soul murder. *The New York Review of Books*, November 8, 1990. http://www.nybooks.com/articles/3458
44. CUBELLS, J. M. and RICART, S., *¿Por qué lloras?* Martínez Roca, Barcelona, 1999.
45. HOLLYER, B. and SMITH, L., *Sleep, the Secret of Problem-free Nights*. Ward Lock, London, 1996.
46. ANDERS, T. F., Night-waking in infants during the first year of life. *Pediatrics*, 1979, 63:860-864.
47. CURELL, N., VIÑALLONGA, X., CUBELLS, J. M., MOLINA,V., ESTIVILL, E., RIOS, J. and LANGUE, J., Dormir amb els pares: prevalença i factors associats en una població de 6 a 36 mesos d'e-dat. *Pediatr. Catalana*, 1999, 59:73-78.
48. LOZOFF, B., ASKEW, G. L. and WOLF, A. W., Cosleeping and early childhood sleep problems: Effects of ethnicity and socioeconomic status. *J. Dev. Behav. Pediatr.*, 1996, 17:9-15.

49. LATZ, S., WOLF, A. W. and LOZOFF, B., Cosleeping in context. Sleep practices and problems in young children in Japan and the United States. *Arch. Pediatr. Adolesc. Med.*, 1999, 153:339–346.

50. GARCIA, A., MALO, J., ISERN, R., JUNCOSA, S., PÉREZ, J. M., RIEROLA, M. and JUVENTENY, D., Es desperten els nens a la nit? *But. Soc. Cat. Pediatr.*, 1995, 55:59.

51. ESTIVILL SANCHO, E., Insomnio infantil. *Act. Ped. Esp.*, 1994, 52:398–401.

52. LOZOFF, B., WOLF, A. W., DAVIS, N. S., Cosleeping in urban families with young children in the United States. *Pediatrics*, 1984, 74:171–182.

53. OKAMI, P., WEISNER ,T. and OLMSTEAD, R., Outcome correlates of parent-child bedsharing: an eighteen-year longitudinal study. *J. Dev. Behav. Pediatr.*, 2002, 23:244–253.

54. FORBES, J. F., WEISS, D. S. and FOLEN, R. A., The cosleeping habits of military children. *Mil. Med.*, 1992, 157:196–200.

55. FAROOQI, S., Ethnic differences in infant care practices and in the incidence of sudden infant death syndrome in Birmingham. *Early Hum Develop.*, 1994, 38:209–213.

56. MOSKO, S., RICHARD, C. and MCKENNA, J., Infant arousals during mother infant bed sharing: implications for infant sleep and sudden infant death syndrome research. *Pediatrics*, 1997, 100:841–849.

57. SCRAGG, R., MITCHELL, E. A., TAYLOR, B. J., STEWART, A., FORD, R. P. K., THOMPSON, J. M. D., ALLEN, E. M. and BECROFT, D. M. O., Bed sharing, smoking, and alcohol in the sudden infant death syndrome. *Br. Med. J.*, 1993, 307:1312–1318.

58. MITCHELL, E. A., TUOHY, P. G., BRUNT, J. M., THOMPSON, J. M. D., CLEMENTS, M. S., STEWART, A. W., FORD, R. P. K. and TAYLOR, B. J., Risk factors for sudden infant death syndrome following the prevention campaign in New Zealand: a prospective study. *Pediatrics*, 1997, 100:835-840.

59. BLAIR, P. S., FLEMING, P. J., SMITH, I. J., PLATT, M. W., YOUNG, J., NADIN, P., BERRY, P. J., GOLDING, J. and the CESDI SUDI RESEARCH GROUP, Babies sleeping with parents: case-control study of factors influencing the risk of the sudden infant death syndrome. *Br. Med. J.*, 1999, 319:1457–1462.

60. SCRAGG, R. K. R., MITCHELL, E. A., STEWART, A. W., FORD, R. P. K., TAYLOR, B. J., HASSALL, I. B., WILLIAMS, S. M. and

THOMPSON, J. M. D., for the New Zealand Cot Death Study Group, Infant room-sharing and prone sleep position in sudden infant death syndrome. *Lancet*, 1996, 347:7–12.

61. WISBORG, K., KESMODEL, U., HENRIKSEN, T. B., OLSEN, S. F. and SECHER, N. J. A., *Prospective study of smoking during pregnancy and SIDS*. Arch. Dis. Child., 2000, 83:203–206.

62. MCKENNA, J. J., MOSKO, S. S. and RICHARD, C. A., Bedsharing promotes breastfeeding. *Pediatrics*, 1997, 100:214–219.

63. PANTLEY, E., *The No-cry Sleep Solution*. Contemporary Books, Chicago, 2002.

64. MALO, J., ISERN, R., GARCÍA GALLEGO, A., JUNCOSA, S., ARMENGOL, P., CABRAL, M., RAMÓN, M. A. and HERNÁNDEZ, V., *Hàbits a l'hora de dormir*. But. Soc. Cat. Pediatr., 1995, 55:45.

65. ROSENFELD, A. A., WENEGRAT, A. O. R., HAAVIK, D. K., WENEGRAT, B. G. and SMITH, C. R., *Sleeping patterns in upper-middleclass families when the child awakens ill or frightened*. Arch. Gen. Psychiatry, 1982, 39:943–947.

66. ADAIR, R., BAUCHNER, H., PHILIPP, B., LEVENSON, S., and ZUCKERMAN, B., *Night waking during infancy: role of parental presence at bedtime*. Pediatrics, 1991, 87:500–504.

67. ADAIR, R., ZUCKERMAN, B., BAUCHNER, H., PHILIPP, B. and LEVENSON, S., *Reducing night waking in infancy: a primary care intervention*. Pediatrics, 1992, 89:585–588.

68. ALETHA SOLTER, *¿Qué hacer cuando un bebé llora?* Aware Parenting Institute. http://www.awareparenting.com/llora.htm

69. NITSCH, C. and SCHELLING, C. von, *Límites a los niños. Cuándo y cómo*. Médici, Barcelona, 1999.

70. BULINGE, P., *La légende picturale napoléonienne dans L'Aiglon d'Edmond Rostand*.

71. SPOCK, B. and ROTHENBERG, M. B., *Baby and Child Care*. Pocket Books, New York, 1985.

72. NICOLAŸ, F., *Los niños mal educados*. Gustavo Gili, Barcelona.

73. SANMARTÍN, J., *Conceptos, tipos e incidencia*. En Sanmartín, J. (ed.): *Violencia contra niños*. Centro Reina Sofía para el Estudio de la Violencia. Ariel, Barcelona, 1999.

74. LESHAN, E., *When Your Child Drives You Crazy*. St. Martin's Press, New York, 1985.

75. FINKELHOR, D., *Victimología infantil*. En Sanmartín, J. (ed.): *Violencia contra niños*. Centro Reina Sofía para el Estudio de la Violencia. Ariel, Barcelona, 1999.

76. GREEN, C., *Toddler taming. A Parents' Guide to the First Four Years*. Vermilion, London, 1992.

77. CASTELLS, P., *Nuestros hijos y sus problemas*. Folio, Barcelona, 1995.

78. CAPA GARCÍA, L., BERCEDO SANZ, A., REDONDO FIGUERO, C., and GONZÁLEZ-ALCITURRI CASANUEVA, M. A., Valoración de la conducta de los niños de Cantabria mediante el cuestionario de Eyberg. *An. Esp. Pediatr.*, 2000, 53:234–240.

79. SAMALIN, N., *Entre el amor y la ira*. Plural, Barcelona, 1993.

80. BOWLBY, J., *The Making and Breaking of Affectional Bonds*. Routledge, 2005.

81. FREUD, S., *Three Essays on the Theory of Sexuality*. Basic Books, 2000.

82. BLANCAFORT, M., *Puericultura actual*. Bruguera, Barcelona, 1979.

83. CHRISTOPHERSEN, E. R., Orientación previsora acerca de la disciplina. *Pedia*, 1986, 4:831–841.

84. BRUER, J. T., *El mito de los tres primeros años*. Paidós, Barcelona, 2000.

85. DILKS, S. A., Developmental aspects of child care. *Pediatr. Clin. N. Amer.*, 1991, 38:1529–1543.

86. WILLINGER M., Ko C. W., HOFFMAN H. J., KESSLER R. C., CORWIN M. J., Trends in Infant Bed Sharing in the United States, 1993-2000. The National Infant Sleep Position Study. *Arch Pediatr Adolesc Med* 2003;157:43–49.

87. CARPENTER, R. G., IRGENS, L. M., BLAIR, P. S., ENGLAND, P. D., FLEMING, P., HUBER, H., JORCH, G., SCHREUDER, P., Sudden unexplained infant death in 20 regions in Europe: case control study. *Lancet* 2004;363:185–191.

88. BLAIR, P. S., SIDEBOTHAM, P., BERRY, P. J., EVANS, M., FLEMING, P. J., Major epidemiological changes in sudden infant death syndrome: a 20-year population-based study in the UK. *Lancet* 2006; 367: 314–319

89. AMERICAN ACADEMY OF PEDIATRICS TASK FORCE ON SUDDEN INFANT DEATH SYNDROME. The changing concept of sudden infant death syndrome: diagnostic coding shifts, controversies regarding the sleeping environment, and new variables to consider in reducing risk. *Pediatrics*, 2005; 116: 1245–1255.

90. BOUCKE, L., El control temprano de los esfínteres. www.

crianzanatural.com/art/art47.html

91. BAUER, I., Diaper free! The gentle wisdom of natural infant hygiene. www.natural-wisdom.com

92. Centro Reina Sofía. Menores víctimas de violencia en el ámbito familiar. http://www.centroreinasofia.es/paneldecontrol/est/pdf/EST009-3270.pdf

93. BRADLEY R. H., VANDELL D. L., Child care and the well-being of children. *Arch. Pediatr. Adolesc. Med.* 2007;161:669–676.

94. American Academy of Pediatrics Committee on Early Childhood, Adoption, and Dependent Care. Quality early education and child care from birth to kindergarten. *Pediatrics*, 2005, 115:187–191.

Index